Otto Meyerhof

The Difficult Life of a Nobel Prize Winner

By

Michael Schmitt

Otto Meyerhof: The Difficult Life of a Nobel Prize Winner

Edited by Michael Schmitt

This book first published 2023

Ethics International Press Ltd, UK

British Library Cataloguing in Publication Data

A catalogue record for this book is available from the British Library

Print Book ISBN: 978-1-80441-245-9

eBook ISBN: 978-1-80441-246-6

Table of Contents

Preface   Werner Arnold... vii

Foreword from the Editor   Michael Schmitt x

Contributors..xii

Chapter 1   Otto Meyerhof: A Researcher's Life Between Fame and
            Expulsion, Michael Schmitt and Avinoam Reichman 1

Chapter 2   Otto Meyerhof: Pioneer of Modern Biochemistry,
            Walter Nickel 25

Chapter 3   Anti-Semitism at Heidelberg University 1933 – 1945,
            Frank Engehausen 37

Chapter 4   Anti-Semitism and Anti-Discrimination in Private Law,
            Marc-Philippe Weller, Greta Göbel and
            Markus Lieberknecht.. 60

Chapter 5   After Halle: Some Thoughts on the Situation of the
            Jewish Community in Germany, Frederek Musall 102

Chapter 6   Judeophobia 2.0 as a Cultural Tradition of Educated Elites:
            Current Anti-Semitism and the Echoes of the Past,
            Monika Schwarz-Friesel.. 109

Chapter 7   Anti-Semitism: The Traps of Definitions,
            Natan Sznaider... 130

Chapter 8   Resurrection of Old Ghosts? 76 years After,
            Michael Wolffsohn 146

Preface

In the year in which we celebrate 1,700 years of Jewish life in Germany, Heidelberg University commemorates the Jewish physician and biochemist Otto Meyerhof, who was awarded the Nobel Prize for Medicine 100 years ago, with a lecture series.

I am very pleased about this, because we should honor the significant cultural contributions made by many Jews in the fine arts, music, literature and science, but we must also always keep in mind the darkest times of these 1700 years, when Jews were persecuted and expelled, cruelly mistreated and murdered in bestial ways. German universities and colleges did not offer any significant resistance to the inhuman ideology of National Socialism and suspended numerous academics from their duties as early as 1933. Respect for the persecuted and murdered Jewish scholars demands that they be remembered.

We owe the initiative for this lecture series to Professor Michael Schmitt of the Medical Faculty of the University of Heidelberg, who in his introductory lecture introduced us to the scientific achievements and the deep humiliations and sufferings of the Jew Otto Meyerhof. A life from the award of the greatest scientific honor, the Nobel Prize, to the revocation of his teaching license and flight to the United States. A life from the award of the greatest scientific honor, the Nobel Prize, to the revocation of his teaching license and his flight to the United States. The life of a man who was an exemplary scientist and showed true human greatness when, after all the atrocities and crimes of the National Socialist dictatorship, he resumed scientific contact with Heidelberg University.

The topic of the expulsion of Jewish scientists during the National Socialist regime touches me very much, because I myself had the opportunity to meet Orientalists in Israel who had managed to escape to Palestine. I would just like to mention the distinguished Arabist and Israel Prize winner Joshua Blau, who recently passed away at the age of 101.

The name Meyerhof is not unknown even to an Orientalist like me. Otto Meyerhof's cousin, Max Meyerhof, was not only a famous ophthalmologist but also a distinguished Arabist. He began his medical studies in Heidelberg, but then continued them in Strasbourg, where he was also able to study Oriental studies with his maternal cousin, the Egyptologist Wilhelm Spiegelberg - a fateful decision. Otto Meyerhof was still a teenager when he took a trip to Egypt with Max Meyerhof. Max must have been so fascinated by the country that he settled there permanently two years later and opened an ophthalmology practice. In addition, he translated medical writings from Arabic and wrote treatises on Arabic medical history. Still in 1932 he received a call to the chair of medical history at the University of Bonn, which he declined because he recognized the danger inherent in the rise of National Socialism. He was thus spared the fate of his cousin Otto. Max died in Egypt and was buried in the Jewish cemetery in Cairo. His works on the history of Arabic medicine were republished in three volumes by the Institute for the History of Arabic-Islamic Sciences at the Johann Wolfgang Goethe University in Frankfurt in 1997.

History is also the field of expertise of Professor Frank Engehausen from the Department of History, whom I had the pleasure of introducing during this ring presentation. One of his main areas of work is the history of National Socialism in regional historical perspectives. With his lecture on anti-Semitism at Heidelberg University from 1933-1945, Frank Engehausen sheds light on the fates of Jewish lecturers and deals with the ousting of Jewish students from the university. He thus places the fate of Otto Meyerhof in a larger context. To have the terrible crimes and atrocities of an inhuman dictatorship like the National Socialist regime as the subject of research is certainly one of the most difficult tasks of a historian.

In my review of Utz Maas's three-volume work on the persecution and emigration of German-speaking linguists from 1933-1945, I wrote: "The psychological stresses to which Maas was subjected in researching this work can be felt in many places," because, according to Maas, "Tracing the persecution forces one to follow in the footsteps of the persecutors."

All contributors to this lecture series therefore deserve our respect for their research and thanks for their contributions published in this volume, which help to preserve the memory of the cruel fates of Jewish scholars under National Socialism.

Prof. Dr. Werner Arnold
Rector
Heidelberg University of Jewish Studies

Foreword by the Editor

100 years ago, Otto Meyerhof was awarded the "Nobel Prize in Physiology or Medicine" for his pioneering work on glycogen metabolism. Otto Meyerhof then suffered a great deal during the National Socialist era. This important topic was also brought to the attention of the general public in view of the current resurgence of anti-Semitism with Heidelberg University's Ruperto Carola Ring Lecture "Otto Meyerhof - A Scientist's Life between Fame and Expulsion" in the summer semester of 2021. Scholars from various disciplines addressed the topic from the perspective of their discipline in the lecture series conceived by the Rectorate and myself. This volume is adapted from the presentations of the respective speakers.[1]

I would like to thank the Rector of the University of Heidelberg, Prof. Dr. Bernhard Eitel, for his support of the content of the lecture series and for providing the necessary funds. I thank the Rector of the Heidelberg University of Jewish Studies (HfJS), Prof. Dr. Werner Arnold, for discussions in the run-up and for his foreword to this volume. My special thanks go to the Meyerhof family, especially to Mr. David Meyerhof, a grandson of Otto Meyerhof, for providing many documents and photographs from the family treasure.

I thank Prof. em. Dr. med. Wolfgang Eckart for his great and important work "The University of Heidelberg under National Socialism" and his tips for the lecture series. Unfortunately, Prof. Eckart has passed away in the meantime, we want to keep a blessed memory of him.

Prof. em. Dr. Eberhard Hofmann and Prof. em. Dr. Renate Ulbrich-Hofmann are to be thanked: as excellent connoisseurs of Otto Meyerhof's life and work, they supported this work with many references and documents in the form of letters and articles.

---

[1] Since the contributions originate from different disciplines, the formal conventions customary there in each case, for example with regard to the structure or the citation method, have been retained.

I would like to thank Prof. Dr. Kai Johnsson, Dr. John Wray and Mr. Herbert Zimmermann for their work on the history of the Max Planck Institute (formerly: the Kaiser Wilhelm Institute) for Medical Research and their dedicated provision of information.

I would like to thank Dr. Ingo Runde, Director of the Archives of Heidelberg University, for providing and digitizing the personal files of Otto Meyerhof and the related documents from the university's Nazi period.

Ms. Monika Conrad and Ms. Fuhrmann-Koch deserve thanks for the excellent organization of this event.

And finally, I sincerely thank all the lecturers who, with passion and commitment, have ventured with me on this exploratory journey through the life of Otto Meyerhof and the aspects of Jewish life in Germany.

We publish this volume in the hope of learning from the past. May memory be a reminder to us to uphold what is good and courageous in people.

Heidelberg, July 2023 / Tammuz 5783

Michael Schmitt
Editor

Contributors

Prof. Dr. Walter Nickel has been conducting research at the Biochemistry Center of Heidelberg University (BZH) since 2000 and has been Professor of Biochemistry at Heidelberg University since 2004. After studying and earning his doctorate at the University of Göttingen, he conducted postdoctoral research at the Memorial Sloan-Kettering Cancer Center in New York City (USA) and at Heidelberg University, where he habilitated in 2001. Since 2019, he has been the Dean of Studies for the Bachelor's and Master's programs in biochemistry at Heidelberg University. Walter Nickel is speaker of the Collaborative Research Center "Molecular Switches in the Space-Time Control of Cellular Signal Transduction" (SFB/ TRR 186 Heidelberg/Berlin) and since 2021 Executive Director of the BZH. His research focuses on the molecular mechanisms for the unconventional secretion of fibroblast growth factor 2 from cancer cells, a process that plays a critical role in tumor-induced angiogenesis. In addition, his research group at BZH is developing novel inhibitors of cellular release of FGF2 that may serve to prevent chemoresistance in the treatment of acute leukemia.

Prof. Dr. Marc-Philippe Weller has been Director at the Institute for Foreign and International Private and Commercial Law at Heidelberg University since 2014. Previously, he studied and received his doctorate in Heidelberg and Montpellier (Licence en droit), habilitated in Cologne (2008) and held chairs at the Universities of Mannheim (2008 - 2011) and Freiburg (2011 - 2014). Visiting professorships in The Hague, Gothenburg, Paris, Taipei, Washington and Vienna, among others. Prorector for International Affairs at Heidelberg University (since 2019). Co-editor of, among others, the Zeitschrift für Unternehmens- und Gesellschaftsrecht (ZGR), the Zeitschrift für Europäisches Privatrecht (ZEuP) and, together with Prof. Dr. Wolfgang Kahl, editor of the Handbuch Climate Change Litigation (2021).

Greta Göbel is a research assistant and dotoral fellow at the Institute for Foreign and International Private and Commercial Law at the University of Heidelberg, Chair of Prof. Dr. Marc-Philippe Weller. Studies at the Ruprecht-Karls-University Heidelberg as well as Université de Lorraine, Nancy (France) (2015-2021).

Dr. Markus Lieberknecht is currently pursuing graduate studies (LL.M.) at Harvard Law School as a Fulbright Scholar and works there as an assistant to Prof. Holger Spamann. Previously, he worked as an attorney in the Dispute Resolution Department at SZA Schilling, Zutt & Anschütz in Mannheim (since 2020, currently on leave of absence), received his doctorate under Prof. Dr. Marc-Philippe Weller at the Institute for Foreign and International Private and Commercial Law at the University of Heidelberg (2018 - 2021), completed his legal clerkship at the Hanseatic Higher Regional Court in Hamburg, Berlin and Karlsruhe (2016 - 2018) and studied in Passau and Istanbul (2009 - 2015).

Prof. Dr. Frank Engehausen teaches Modern History at the Department of History of Heidelberg University. His work focuses on 19th and 20th century German history; he has published on the 1848/49 Revolution, National Socialism, Southwest German regional history, and the history of Heidelberg University, among other topics. He is a member of the Commission for Historical Regional Studies in Baden-Württemberg. In 2006 and 2007, Engehausen investigated the "History of the Josefine and Eduard von Portheim Foundation for Science and Art 1919-1955" on behalf of the University and the City of Heidelberg, and from 2014 to 2017 he coordinated the research project "History of the State Ministries in Baden and Württemberg during the National Socialist era." Currently, his book "Tatort Heidelberg. Everyday Stories of Repression and Persecution 1933-1945" was published.

Professor Dr. Michael Wolffsohn is one of the leading experts on the analysis of international politics and not least the relations between Germans and Jews on the state, political, economic and religious levels. The historian and publicist regularly speaks out on important political, military, historical and religious issues. On topics such as the future of the Bundeswehr, the Middle East and other world conflicts, German-Israeli relations, or the history and present of Judaism, he has made a name for himself with precise analyses and clear statements. He was Professor of Modern History at the University of the Federal Armed Forces in Munich from 1981-2012 and received, among other honors, the Order of Merit of the Federal Republic of Germany in 1988. Prof. Dr. Michael Wolffsohn was historian and publicist, and university lecturer of the year 2017, books with including "Deutschjüdische Glückskinder" (as a children's and young people's book in 2021), "Tacheles", "Zum Weltfrieden".

Prof. Dr. Natan Sznaider, born in Mannheim in 1954 as the child of stateless survivors of the Shoah from Poland, went to Israel at the age of 20 and studied sociology, psychology and history at the University of Tel Aviv. In 1984, he received his doctorate from Columbia University in New York with a thesis entitled "The Social History of Compassion." He is a retired professor of sociology at the Tel Aviv Academic College. Most recently published: Vanishing Points of Memory. On the Presence of the Holocaust and Colonialism. Hanser, 2022.

Prof. Dr. Frederek Musall studied Jewish Studies, Islamic/Arabic Studies, Semitic Studies and Comparative Religion in Heidelberg and Jerusalem. He received his PhD in 2005 from Prof. Dr. Yossef Schwartz (Tel Aviv University) and Prof. Dr. Raif Georges Khoury, (Ruprecht-Karls-Universität Heidelberg) on the two medieval Jewish philosophers Moses Maimonides and Chasdai Kreskas. From 2015 till 2023 he was Associate Professor (W2) of Jewish philosophy and intellectual history at the Heidelberg University of Jewish Studies. In the summer semester of 2016, he was Visiting Professor and Deputy Executive Director of the Institute for Jewish Studies at Martin Luther University Halle-Wittenberg. At the beginning of the summer semester 2017, he was appointed Deputy Rector of the Heidelberg University of Jewish Studies. In 2023 he was appointed as a Full Professor (W3) for Jewish Studies at the Würzburg University. His research interests include philosophical, theological, and mystical

Jewish traditions of thought (especially in its multiple relations to corresponding Arab-Islamic traditions of thought), processes of Jewish identity formation, Jewish popular culture, and methodology in Jewish Studies. His most recent publication is "And at last we could talk ..." Eine Handreichung zu jüdisch-muslimischem Dialog in der Praxis, Freiburg: Herder 2020.

Prof. Dr. Michael Schmitt has been Siebeneicher Endowed Professor for Cellular Immunotherapy and Head of the GMP Laboratory for Cell Product and Vaccine Manufacturing at Heidelberg University, Germany, since 2011. He studied Medicine and Oriental Studies at Saarland University in Homburg, Germany with semesters abroad at Tel-Aviv University and Harvard Medical School, Boston, USA. 1992 PhD with Prof. Richard Berberich on iron metabolism and erythrocytes. Then research stay 1994-98 in Japan with Prof. H. Shiku on topics of tumor vaccination. Specialist in internal medicine, hematology, oncology and clinical infectiology and habilitation on immunogenic leukemia antigens at the University of Ulm. At the University of Rostock 2009-2011 head of stem cell transplantation. 1999 Novartis Research Prize, 2005 Felix Skubiszewski Medal of the Medical University of Lublin and 2008 Hans-Jochen-Illiger Memorial Prize. Part of Michael Schmitt's research group conducts research in the laboratories of the Otto Meyerhof Center (OMZ), which was founded by Heidelberg University in 2001.

Dr. Avinoam Reichman began his studies in General and Comparative Literature at the University of Frankfurt and eventually switched to studying human medicine at the Justus Liebig University of Giessen. After graduating in 2020, he completed his PhD under Prof. Michael Schmitt at Heidelberg University Hospital on the topic of "Cellular Immunotherapy". During his studies, he completed numerous stays at Israeli Torah schools (Yeshivot) in Tel Aviv and Jerusalem, among other places. He is currently working as a resident at the University Hospital of Regensburg.

Prof. Monika Schwarz-Friesel is a cognitive scientist and antisemitism researcher. She is head of the Department of Language and Communication at the Technical University of Berlin. Her empirical research focusses on both historical and contemporary manifestations of Jew hatred, the Israelization of antisemitism and on the emotional basis of antisemitism. Her latest research projects deal with Jew- hatred on the internet 2.0, and most recently with the re-traumatization in the third generation of Jews in Germany. She has published several books on antisemitism, among them *"Inside the Antisemitic Mind"*, with Jehuda Reinharz, 2017, Boston, USA. She is Member of the Advisory Board for Antisemitism Studies (USA) and the scientific board of the *Journal of Contemporary Antisemitism* (UK), as well as Chair of the board of trustees of the Rabbiner-Leo-Trepp-Stiftung.

Chapter One

Otto Meyerhof: A Researcher's Life Between Fame and Expulsion

Michael Schmitt and Avinoam Reichman

100 years ago, Otto Meyerhof was awarded the Nobel Prize for Medicine, which he then received in 1922 for his pioneering work on glycogen metabolism. Otto Meyerhof suffered a great deal during the National Socialist era. In view of the current resurgence of anti-Semitism, this important topic is being brought to the attention of the general public with the Ruperto Carola Lecture Series at Heidelberg University, "Otto Meyerhof - A Scientist's Life between Fame and Expulsion" this summer semester. Scientists from various disciplines addressed the topic from the perspective of their discipline in the lecture series conceived by the Rectorate and Prof. Schmitt. This volume contains the lectures

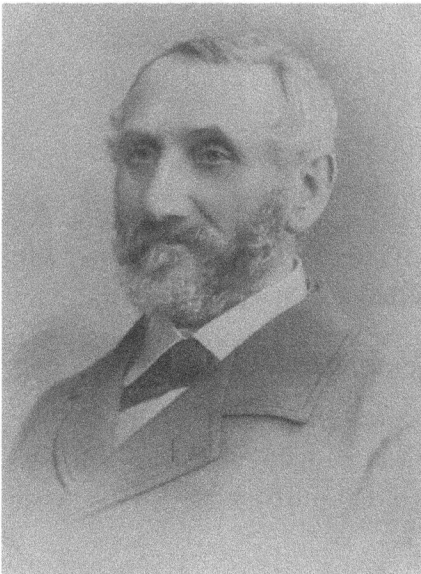

Figure 1: Israel Meyerhof, 1811-1855

of the respective speakers, in a form written down by them. In the hope of reviving the past in the present, the memory serves as a vigil to uphold the good and the courage in human beings.

The Meyerhofs were established textile merchants in Hildesheim since the beginning of the 18th century. Israel Meyerhof (1811-1885) (Fig. 1), Otto Meyerhof's paternal grandfather, was a "white goods", i.e. textile merchant[1]. Like so many of his contemporaries, he ventured the step from manufactory to industrialization.[1] His products consisted of "Barchent" products, a textile mixture of linen and cotton.[1] Due to him, the family left Hildesheim, which had been inhabited since the 18th century, to finally settle in Berlin via an intermediate stay in Hanover.[1] Israel Meyerhof was still firmly integrated into the social structures of his Jewish fellow citizens at that time. He was regularly involved in the synagogue community. His father Isaak Meyerhof had set up a foundation for poorer schoolchildren from Jewish families.[1]

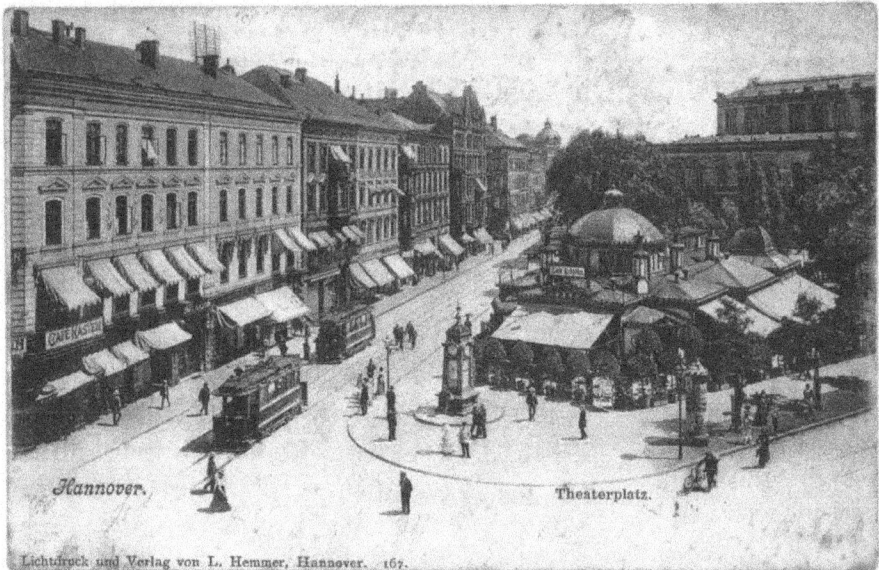

Figure 2: Otto Meyerhof's birthplace

Israel Meyerhof's son, Felix Meyerhof (1849-1923), then moved with his wife Bettina Meyerhof, née Mai (1862-1915), to what would later become Otto Meyerhof's birthplace, near the Opera House next to today's Cafe Kröpcke (Fig. 2).[1] Otto Meyerhof (1884-1951) and his siblings Therese (1882-1971) and Walter (1886-1930) (Figs. 3 + 4)[1], were born there. Felix Meyerhof then moved to Berlin with his family and Otto, who was four years old at the time, to run the newly

---

[1] Selke, W. and C. Heppner (2017). The family of the Nobel Laureate Otto Meyerhof in Hannover, in book: Hannoversche Geschichtsblaetter 71 (2017), pp. 156-166.

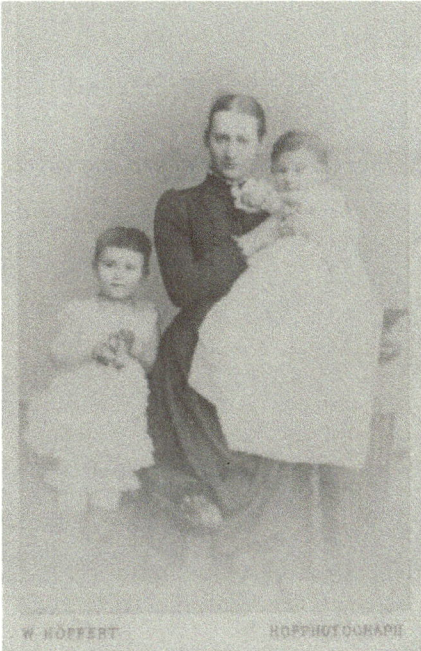

Figure 3: Bettina Meyerhof,
with her children Therese and Otto,
in November 1884.

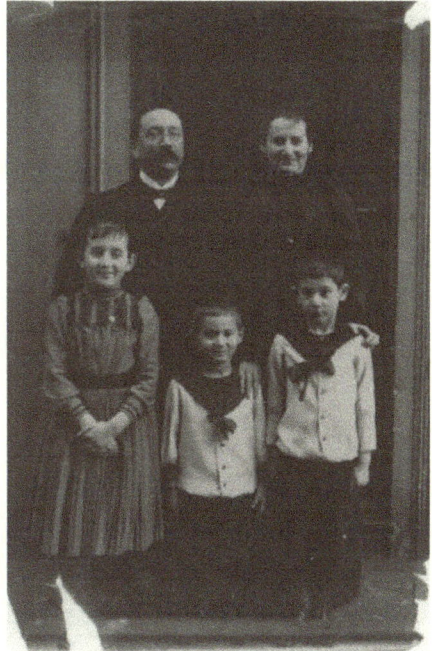

Figure 4: Felix and Bettina Meyerhof,
with their children Therese, Otto
and Karl, in 1890.

founded company I. Meyerhof, a manufactory goods store, with his siblings. There, Otto Meyerhof prepared for university during his school years.[3] Already as a teenager he fell ill with a chronic kidney disease, which confined him to bed at an early age and gave him the opportunity to study philosophy and especially the literature of Goethe. From then on, Goethe's writings, poetry and work on natural research accompanied him throughout his life. Meyerhof said about Goethe's scientific work, especially about "The Theory of colors", that it was not an exact science, nor did he want it to be. It was not the creation of a natural scientist, but of a nature lover. Goethe himself had said that he was not interested in grasping the world mathematically and physically.[2]

Due to Otto's many stays in several cure centers, the family decided, among other things, that Otto should travel to the Nile together with his cousin Dr. Max Meyerhof (Fig. 5), physician and Egyptologist.[3] Max Meyerhof was fluent in Arabic and was highly regarded by the locals as the ophthalmologist "Dr. Max".[2] He eventually became vice president of the local Ophthalmological Society, vice president of the German Archaeological Institute in Cairo, and continued to write

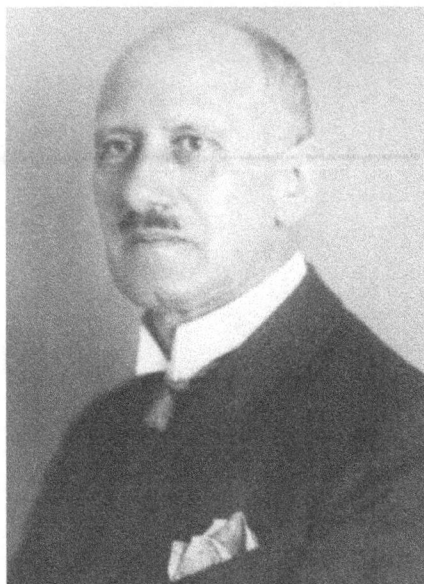

Figure 5: Max Meyerhof (1874- 1945)

orientalist, largely historical, works on Arabic medicine and pharmacology. He translated for example the text "The Ten Treatises on the Eye," written around the 9th century by Hunain Ibn Is-Haq (808-873), from Arabic into English.[3] In 1945, Max Meyerhof was buried in the Ashkenazi synagogue in Cairo. Otto Meyerhof, who was affected by that travel throughout his life, was newly interested in archaeology and Islamic art, and had a strong commitment to patients living in poverty, inspired by his cousin. He graduated from high school in Berlin in 1903 and began studying medicine and philosophy at the universities of Berlin, Strasbourg, and Heidelberg afterwards.[3] In Berlin, he met Leonard Nelson (Fig. 6), who later became a professor of philosophy in Göttingen.[4]

---

[2] Hofmann E (2016) Otto Warburg und Otto Meyerhof – die Geschichte einer Freundschaft BIOspektrum 6:662-664

[3] Hofmann E (2016) Otto Meyerhof – Humanist und Naturforscher: Von der Philosophie zum Nobelpreis. Acta Historica Leopoldina 65:299–369

[4] Ekkehard H. Theodor Lessing – Otto Meyerhof – Leonard Nelson – Bedeutende Juden in Niedersachsen, Niedersächsische Landeszentrale für politische Bildung, 1964

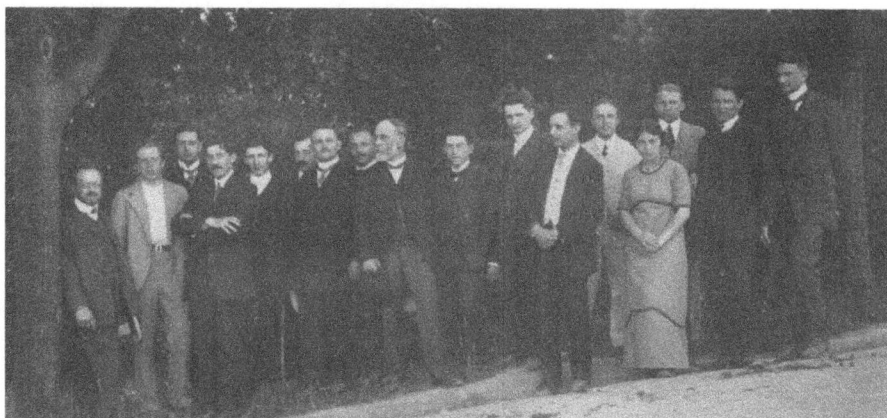

Figure 6: The "New Friesian School" of philosophy with Leonard Nelson (2nd from left) and Otto Meyerhof (4th from left). The only lady is Hedwig Schallenberg who married Otto later.

Leonard Nelson's philosophy was based on Kant's critique of reason. He dealt with the criticism by, and a critical handling of reason with itself. Nelson's primary interest continued to be the formation of the foundations of an ethics that makes it possible to consider the interests of the parties in conflict through dialogue. Thus, he extended Kant's Categorical Imperative to include the experiential world of the individual. Nelson's understanding of philosophy was strongly influenced by the Socratic teaching method. It was central not to indoctrinate students with facts, but to encourage them to think for themselves.[2]

He had a lifelong friendship with Nelson, which was expressed in intensive correspondence between the two. Through Nelson, Meyerhof was introduced to philosophy. A few years later, he also acted as a mediator between a philosophical dispute between Nelson and the New Kantian Ernst Cassirer.[2] The writings of Immanuel Kant and Jakob Friedrich Fries were of particular interest to the young students. Thus, Leonard Nelson founded the New Friesian School in 1903.[2] Representatives of different disciplines, mathematicians, physicians, and philosophers met there regularly in Göttingen to exchange ideas on philosophical topics.[2] Hedwig Schallenberg also met Otto Meyerhof there. They married in 1914 (Fig. 7).

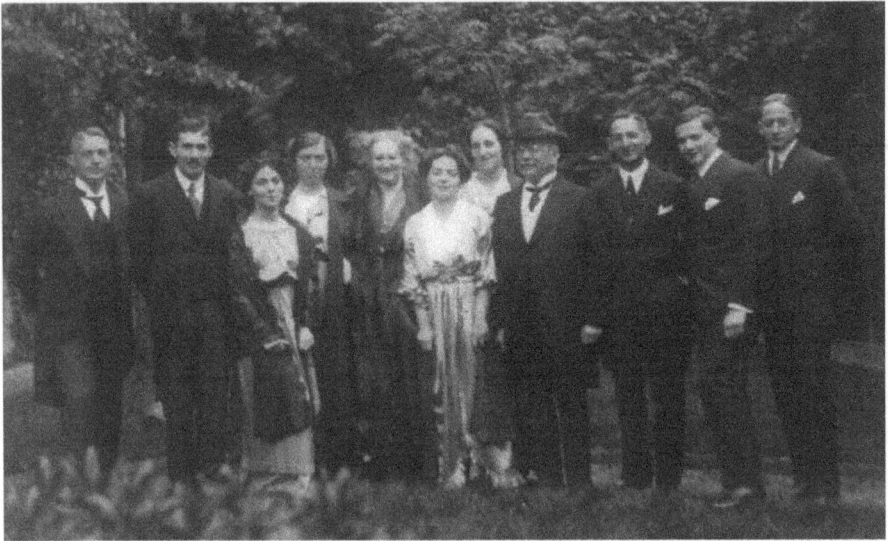

Figure 7: Wedding of Otto (2nd from left) und Hedwig (3rd from left), Hedwig's mother (5th from left) and her sister and father (6th and 7th from left)

Meyerhof and Nelson were not primarily interested in politics, but they were socially engaged. Even as students at Berlin University, they gave evening classes for workers.[2] This was intended not only to improve the education of the working class, but also to awaken in the students a sense of social obligation in order to alleviate social antagonisms. The authorities of the time viewed this commitment as questionable: "It was likely to seduce students into indolence in their studies." Thus, in 1922, the Westphalian daily newspaper "die Glocke" headlined an article on Meyerhof's receipt of the Nobel Prize with the title: "The industrious Nobel Prize winner. "[3] Despite this supposed industriousness, Otto Meyerhof finally passed his state examination in medicine with the grade 1.

After a stay in Strasbourg in 1905, where Otto studied Goethe's writings on natural research, especially the theory of colors, Meyerhof finally arrived in Heidelberg in 1907 as a medical student and doctor for the poor. There Meyerhof met the psychiatrist and psychoanalyst Arthur Kronfeld (1886-1941), as well as the physiologist Viktor von Weizsäcker (1886 - 1957), the Jewish cell physiologist and biochemist Otto Warburg (1883 - 1970), with whom he was to remain in friendship throughout his life, and the philosopher Karl Jaspers (1883 - 1969).

He wrote his dissertation thesis (Fig. 8) with Ludolf von Krehl (1861-1937), which was partly influenced by this circle of people, around 1910 under the title: "Contributions to the Psychological Theory of Mental Disorders."

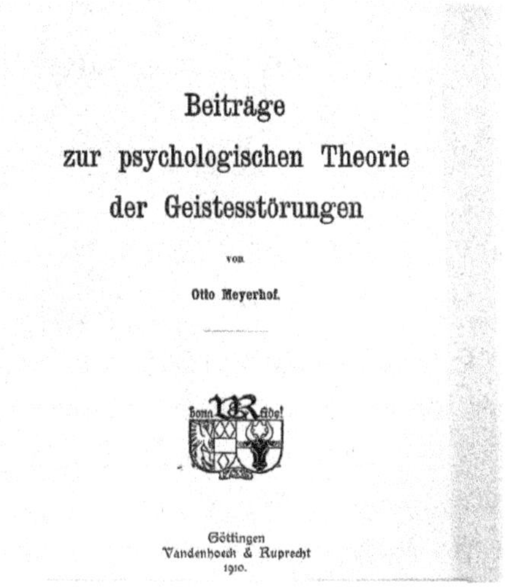

Beiträge

zur psychologischen Theorie

der Geistesstörungen

von

Otto Meyerhof.

Göttingen
Vandenhoeck & Ruprecht
1910.

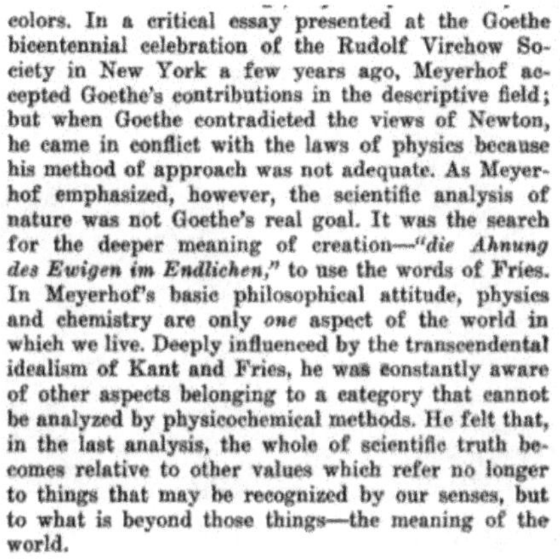

colors. In a critical essay presented at the Goethe bicentennial celebration of the Rudolf Virchow Society in New York a few years ago, Meyerhof accepted Goethe's contributions in the descriptive field; but when Goethe contradicted the views of Newton, he came in conflict with the laws of physics because his method of approach was not adequate. As Meyerhof emphasized, however, the scientific analysis of nature was not Goethe's real goal. It was the search for the deeper meaning of creation—"*die Ahnung des Ewigen im Endlichen*," to use the words of Fries. In Meyerhof's basic philosophical attitude, physics and chemistry are only *one* aspect of the world in which we live. Deeply influenced by the transcendental idealism of Kant and Fries, he was constantly aware of other aspects belonging to a category that cannot be analyzed by physicochemical methods. He felt that, in the last analysis, the whole of scientific truth becomes relative to other values which refer no longer to things that may be recognized by our senses, but to what is beyond those things—the meaning of the world.

Figure 8: Otto Meyerhof's Dissertation, Contributions to the Psychological Theory of Mental Disorders 1910

Figure 9: Obituary by Severo Ochoa

An obituary in the journal Science in 1951 of Meyerhof's later student and Nobel laureate Severo Ochoa (fig. 9) says: "It was the search for deeper meaning of creation-"the presentiment of the eternal in the finite," to use the words of Fries. "In Meyerhof's basic philosophical attitude, physics and chemistry are only one aspect of the world in which we live." This holistic or integrated view of the world shaped Otto's entire life and work.

Otto Meyerhof met Otto Warburg (Fig. 10) while he was still a student in Heidelberg. He accompanied Warburg to Naples in 1911 for a research stay at the local Zoological Station. Both later worked together for several years at the Kaiser Wilhelm Institute for Biology in Berlin-Dahlem (Fig. 11).[5] Warburg's father was also of Jewish descent and at the time a physics professor in Freiburg im Breisgau and president of the Physikalisch-Technische-Reichsanstalt

[5] Hofmann E (2016) Otto Warburg und Otto Meyerhof – die Geschichte einer Freundschaft BIOspektrum 6:662-664

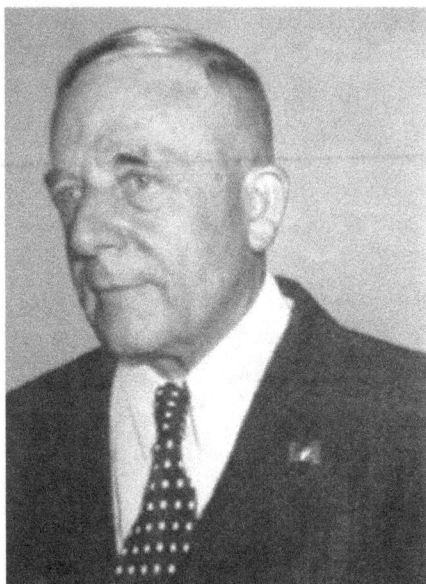

Figure 10: Otto Warburg (1883-1970)

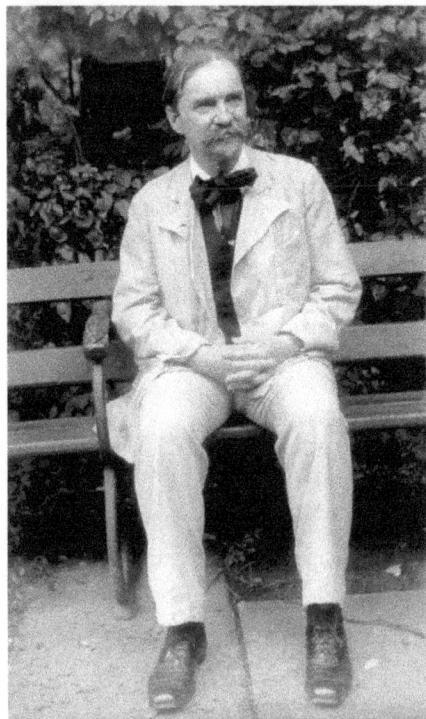

Figure 11: Kaiser Wilhelm Institute for Biology in Berlin-Dahlem, 1940.

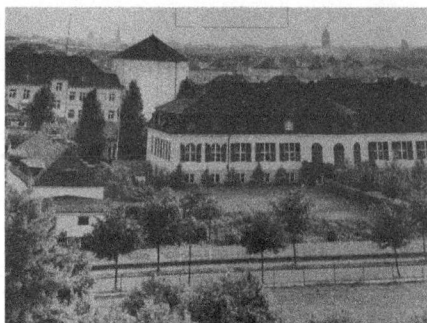

Figure 12: Ludolf von Krehl
(1861- 1937)

in Berlin. Thus Warburg already got to know the great scientists of his time at home, including Albert Einstein, Emil Fischer, Walther Nernst and Max Planck. Otto Warburg received his doctorate under Ludolf von Krehl "On oxidation in living cells after experiments on the sea urchin egg (Fig. 12)." As early as 1912, he became head of department at the Kaiser Wilhelm Institute of Biology in Berlin-Dahlem. There, too, his main interest remained the study of biological oxidation-reduction processes (see chapter 2 by W. Nickel). Otto Meyerhof, inspired by Warburg's work on sea urchin eggs, first began his own marine biological work. At this time, his gradual detachment from philosophy occurred in favor of experimental natural history

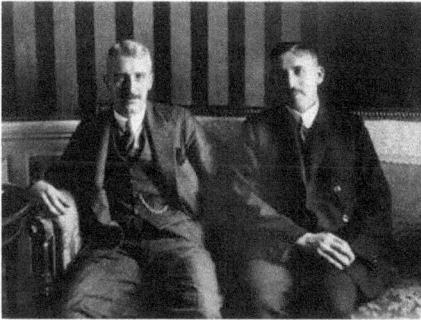

Figure 13: Archibald Vivian Hill (1886-1977), with Otto Meyerhof

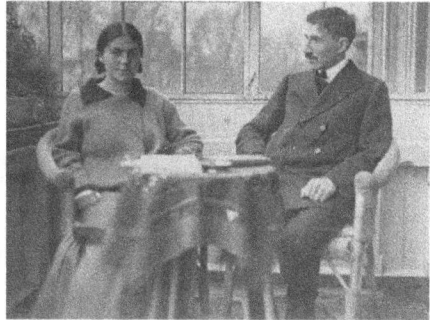

Figure 14: Otto and Hedwig Meyerhof in Kiel

research.[6] In return for his friend Warburg, however, Meyerhof was only granted an unpaid assistantship at the Physiological Institute of Kiel University in 1912, where he habilitated in 1913.[7] In 1922, Otto Meyerhof, together with Archibald Vivian Hill (1886-1977) (Fig. 13), received the Nobel Prize in Physiology/Medicine for their research on the physiology of muscle and, in particular, the relationship between oxygen consumption and lactic acid production in muscle.[8] In the same year, the Jewish physiologist and mentor of Meyerhof, Rudolf Höber (1873-1953), established a new chair for physiological chemistry in the Physiological Institute of the Medical Faculty in Kiel and proposed Otto Meyerhof for it. This was followed by a discriminatory rejection on the part of the Institute on the grounds that "Höber was already a Jew".[9] Thus, the deeply offended 38-year-old Otto Meyerhof, who had just been awarded the Nobel Prize, remained a private lecturer in an assistant position at the Kiel Institute (Fig. 14). Mediated by Otto Warburg, among others, Meyerhof finally received a position as director of the Kaiser Wilhelm

---

[6] Hofmann E (2016) Otto Warburg und Otto Meyerhof – die Geschichte einer Freundschaft BIOspektrum 6:662-664

[7] Hofmann E (2016) Otto Warburg und Otto Meyerhof – die Geschichte einer Freundschaft BIOspektrum 6:662-664

[8] The Nobel Prize in Physiology or Medicine 1922. NobelPrize.org. Nobel Prize Outreach AB 2021. Sun. 27 Jun 2021. <https://www.nobelprize.org/prizes/medicine/1922/summary/>

[9] Eckart, W. U., et al. (2006). Die Universität Heidelberg im Nationalsozialismus, Springer Berlin Heidelberg.

Institute (KWI) for Medical Research in Heidelberg.[10] The Kaiser Wilhelm Society (KWG) created new institutes for basic medical research as early as the 1920s. For example, the KWG negotiated a plan to establish an institute in "Heidelberg for the entire field of experimental medicine, in which in particular the border areas between medicine, physiology, chemistry and physics should be researched".[11] The Baden government agreed to incorporate the new institute in Heidelberg into the Institute for Experimental Cancer Research. This had been founded in 1906 by Vincenz Czerny (1842-1916). The decision to found the Heidelberg KWI was taken in 1927, and the inauguration of the new building designed by the architect Hans Freese took place three years later (Fig. 15), at the end of May 1930 (Fig. 16). After the occupation of the institute by American troops in March 1945, it was incorporated and renamed the "Max Planck Institute (MPI) for Medical Research" in 1948.[11]

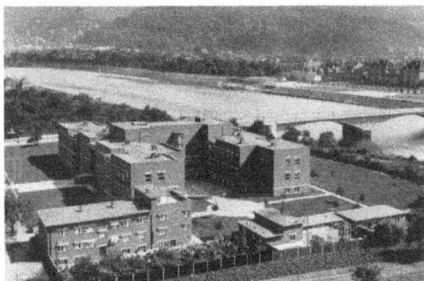

Figure 15: Kaiser-Wilhelm Institute in Heidelberg

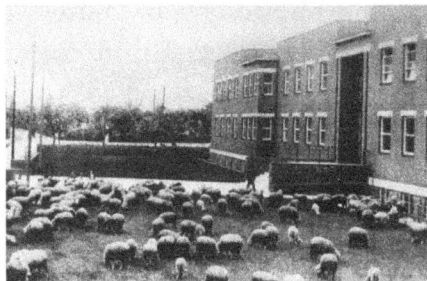

Figure 16: Kaiser-Wilhelm Institute in Heidelberg, 1930.

The time in Heidelberg was very pleasant and productive for Otto Meyerhof. It was also during this time that he wrote one of Meyerhof's major works, „Die Chemischen Vorgänge im Muskel und ihr Zusammenhang mit Arbeitsleistung und Wärmebildung. In this book, Meyerhof pays special tribute to the contributions and achievements of his student Karl Lohmann (1898-1978), discoverer of adenosine triphosphate (ATP) (see Chapter 2 by W. Nickel).

---

[10] Eckart, W.U. Max-Planck-Institut für medizinische Forschung Heidelberg, Denkorte, Max-Planck-Gesellschaft und Kaiser-Wilhelm-Gesellschaft; Brüche und Kontinuitäten; 1911 - 2011 Dresden: Sandstein-Verl., 2010.

In 1991, Gottfried Meyerhof summarized his father's time in Heidelberg as follows[11]: *"My father had very regular and sedate habits. In the twenties and thirties he usually got up at about half past eight in the morning and then had breakfast, usually reading the newspaper, after the children had already gone to school. Around ten o'clock he went to the institute on foot, or in Heidelberg often by bicycle, and came home at one o'clock for lunch with the family. Because of a sensitive stomach, he was given a light diet, with which he enjoyed red wine. He then took a nap with a black bandage over his eyes. After a then enjoyable tea, he went back to the Institute about half past three in the afternoon, where he worked until about half past five. After dinner with the family, he retired to his study at home [...]."* It continues, *"He almost always wrote his papers and letters by hand; the manuscripts were put on paper in pencil so that they could be more easily improved, before he dictated them to his private secretary at the Institute. He rarely typed letters himself at home, and always answered his correspondences promptly. Of his publications, which averaged almost monthly during his forty years of scientific activity, he wrote many in the name of his collaborators, so that they too would have their right to publication. He decided himself on the employment of his collaborators, from whom he always demanded handwritten applications so that they could be examined by a friend and graphologist with regard to personal characteristics. [...]. With the same intentions, Max Planck, the president of the Kaiser Wilhelm Society, and other influential scientists also came to our house at that time for talks, which were usually conducted with the shutters down and in a low voice, during which I was occasionally allowed to offer cigarettes, but then had to leave the room as quickly as possible. [...] A very liberal man, he voted for the Social Democrats; he was a pacifist and a member of the International Rotary Club. Like many others, he initially believed that the political turnaround of 1933 would last only a short time. He often emphasized that at no other place he would get such a professionally satisfying place to work with such reliable and capable scientific and technical staff in an institute set up entirely according to his wishes as in Heidelberg."*

---

[11] Prof. Dr. Gottfried Meyerhof, Erinnerung an das Leben von Otto Meyerhof in Deutschland; Naturwissenschaftliche Rundschau, Heft 10; 44. Jahrg., 1991.

In March 1933, a momentous break in Germany's history occurred with the seizure of power by the National Socialists under their leader Adolf Hitler.[12]

Hitler transformed Germany into a dictatorship, bringing all areas of public life into line according to the Führer principle. Thus, on April 5, 1933, two days before the "Reich Law for the Restoration of the Professional Civil Service," the "Baden Decree on Jews" was published.[13] It was the first decree to "suspend all Jews in public service. Under the pretext of a "strong disturbance of the population" it was ordered that "for the protection and in the interest" of the Jews of Baden all state employees "of the Jewish race" be granted leave until further notice. On April 7, 1933, the order was carried out by the Reich Law for the Restoration of the Professional Civil Service: "(§3) Civil servants and employees of 'non-Aryan descent' shall be retired or lose their teaching credentials, unless they or their fathers had been participants in the war or had been in state service without interruption since August 1, 1914)." "Non-Aryan" descent, according to this law, meant descent from at least one Jewish grandparent, without regard to whether they converted to Christianity or not. As a result of this law, 21 professors, private lecturers and lecturers had to leave the university in Heidelberg.[17] There were also moderate voices against the decision of April 5: Dean Richard Siebeck (Fig. 17) declared the planned dismissals

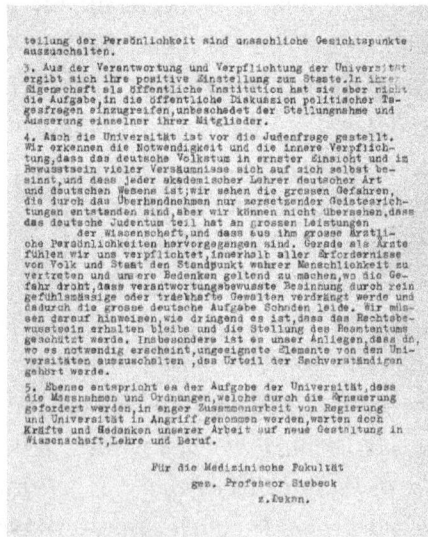

Figure 17: Letter from the Dean, Richard Siebeck

[12] Fest, J. (1973). Hitler: eine Biographie, Ullstein. S.533ff.

[13] Dörflinger G (2012), Juden an der Universität Heidelberg Dokumente aus sieben Jahrhunderten, Ruprecht-Karls-Universität Heidelberg Universitätsbibliothek – Ausstellungen < http://www.tphys.uni heidelberg.de/Ausstellung/>

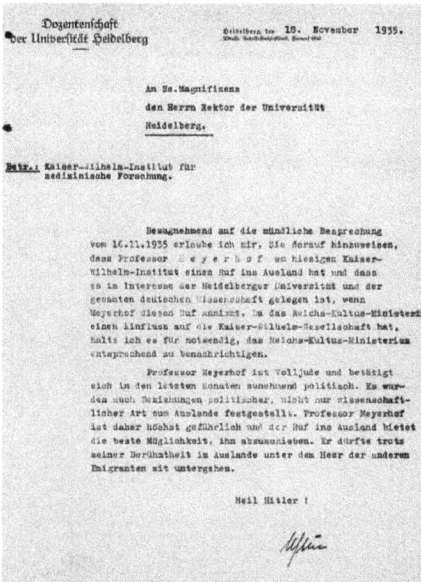

Figure 18: Letter from Assistant Professor Hermann Schlüter to the Rector Wilhelm Groh, 1935

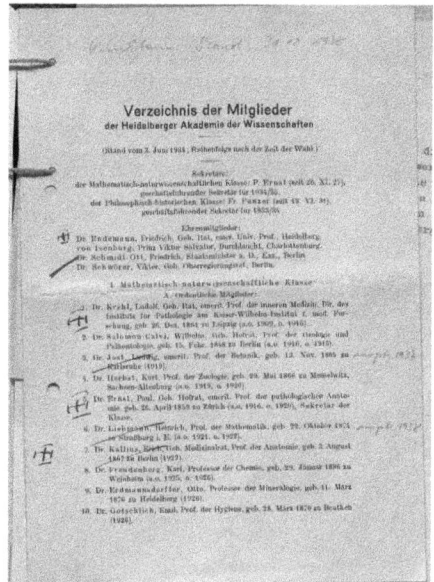

Figure 19: List of University professors dismissed by December 31, 1935

of Jewish academics to be an "encroachment on the self-government of the universities and the civil service law."[14] Acknowledging the existence of a "Jewish question," Siebeck, a physician, called for "state action in the spirit of true humanity," referring to the "great scientific achievements of German Jewry." The letter, however, had no effect on the addressee, the Ministry of Culture. Meyerhof was personally involved for the first time in a letter dated November 18, 1935, from the head of the faculty, a resident named Hermann Schlüter (Fig. 18) to the then Rector Wilhelm Groh regarding an appointment of Meyerhof abroad: "Professor Meyerhof is a full Jew and is becoming increasingly politically active. Relations of a political and not only scientific nature with foreign countries have also been established. Professor Meyerhof is therefore highly dangerous and the appointment abroad offers the best opportunity to get rid of him." A list from the Rectorate (Fig. 19) of university professors dismissed by December 31, 1935 included, among others, the then honorary citizen and geologist Salomon Calvi (1868-1941) (see Chapter 3 by Frank Engehausen).

---

[14] Universitätsarchiv Heidelberg

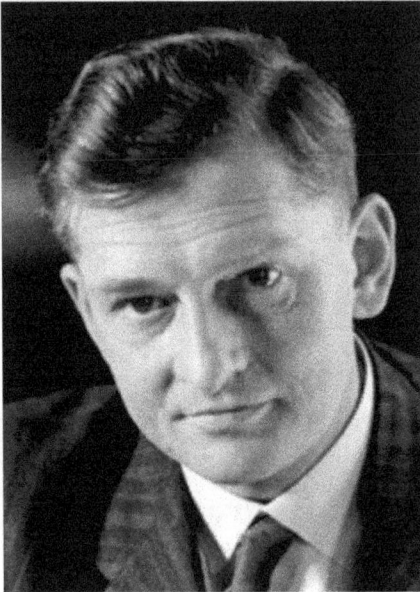

Figure 20: Richard Kuhn (1900 – 1967)

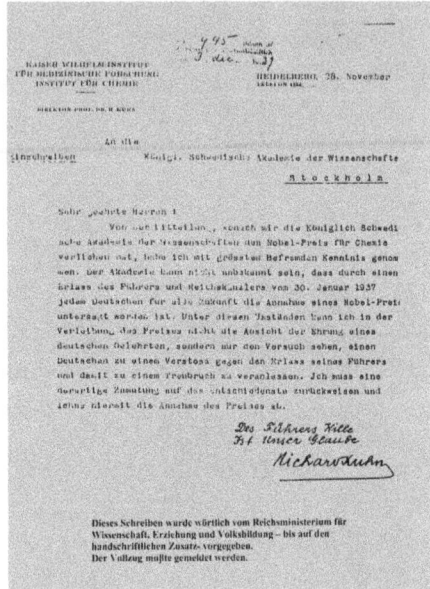

Figure 22: Letter from Richard Kuhn to the Nobel Academy in Stockholm

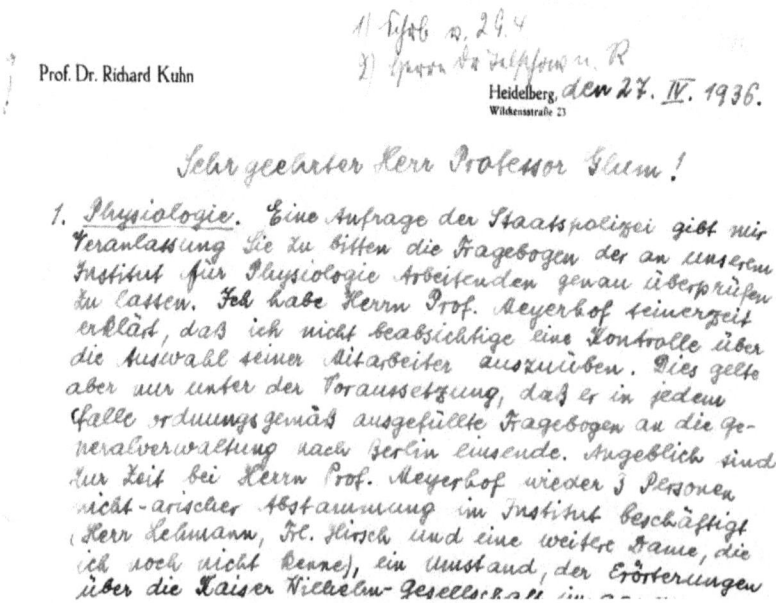

Figure 21: Letter from Richard Kuhn, 1936

Otto Meyerhof was one of the four founding directors, along with von Krehl (pathology), Karl Wilhelm Hausser (physics) and Kuhn (chemistry), honorary professor at the university. One of his three colleagues in the directorate of KWI was Richard Kuhn (1900-1967) (Fig. 20), Nobel laureate in chemistry. Kuhn became department director of chemistry at the KWI for Medical Research in 1930. He lived as Otto Meyerhof's neighbor at Wilckensstr. 23 in Heidelberg. In 1937, after the death of Ludolf von Krehl, Kuhn took over the overall direction of the Institute. As a denunciation in 1936, Kuhn wrote in a letter to the general administration of the Kaiser Wilhelm Society in Berlin: *"Allegedly, three persons of non-Aryan descent are again employed at present by Prof. Meyerhof in the Institute (Mr. Lehmann, Miss Hirsch, and another lady whom I do not yet know)* (Fig. 21)." In 1938, Kuhn received a call for the Nobel Prize in Chemistry for his research on carotenoids and vitamins from the Swedish Committee and rejected it, due to the ban at that time by the government and its leader Adolf Hitler. Kuhn signed the rejection with the words, "The Führer's will is our faith (Fig. 22)." Three years after the end of World War II, he finally accepted the Nobel Prize in 1948. During wartime from 1939-1945, Kuhn worked on poison gas research and was a co-investigator on human experiments at the Heidelberg Tuberculosis Sanatorium, as well as at the Natzweiler concentration camp. In 1948 he became director of the now renamed Max Planck Institute for Medical Research. In 1950, he became a full professor at the University of Heidelberg. In 1951, Kuhn met Otto Meyerhof in Philadelphia; the following night, Otto Meyerhof died of a second heart attack. "Kuhn's career, meanwhile, continued to develop: he became vice president of the Max Planck Society in 1959 and president of the Society of German Chemists in 1964. "18 "After his death in 1967, BASF inaugurated a medal in his honor. "18 It was not until 2005, after the publication on Kuhn's life by Ute Deichmann, that the award was discontinued.

Ute Deichmann writes in her "Statement on his political behaviour during the time of the National Socialists with respect to the question: Can we declare that Kuhn was a role model for chemists?":[15]

> "Meyerhof, who emigrated to France after his release in 1938, from there during the war via Spain and Portugal to the USA (Philadelphia), formulated a long letter to Kuhn on 1.11.1946 (it contains the note: "not sent"), from which excerpts are quoted below. Meyerhof was not informed about all details of Kuhn's activities during the Nazi period, (e.g., he did not know about his combat gas research). *"It is not easy for me, after all the events of the last few years, to write to you openly in the spirit of our old comradeship and thereby to take a stand on the serious question you raise in your second letter. ... I acknowledge with gratitude that by preserving my group of co-workers, by keeping my former institute and my villa free, you took precautions to keep my return to Heidelberg open after the end of the Nazi reign of terror. However, I cannot be content with this recognition. In exchange for the loss of my old place of work, all my possessions and the temporary threat to my existence, I have now at least exchanged the advantages of freedom and self-determination, while you spent this time in a secure position and the ability to work, but in the moral nitrogen air of the Third Reich. This alone does not separate us, and I do not blame anyone for making compromises in order to maintain office and place of work. But you yourself went far beyond that. I cannot conceal the criticism levelled at you by your colleagues in the Allied countries for having voluntarily placed your admirable scientific achievement and chemical mastery in the service of a regime of whose unspeakable vileness and wickedness you were well aware. This was particularly painful to me myself, because I knew in what liberal spirit you had grown up and how this corresponded to your dispositions and nature."*

---

[15] Memento vom 11. Dezember 2007 https://web.archive.org/web/20071211082823/ http://www.gdch.de/oearbeit/deich_kuhn.pdf : Richard Kuhn, 1900-1967, Stellungnahme zu seinem politischen Verhalten während der NS-Zeit unter der Fragestellung: Kann Kuhn als Persönlichkeit Vorbildcharakter in der Chemie zuerkannt werden

In 1947, the American military government in Heidelberg demanded an expert opinion on Kuhn from Meyerhof. In it Meyerhof wrote:

"... Professor Kuhn is an apolitical person. He enjoyed a liberal education, held democratic views during the Weimar Republic, and was a faithful and loyal student of the famous German-Jewish chemist R. Willstätter. Notwithstanding this fact, he acquiesced with the Nazi regime on a number of key issues. Apparently after I had lost my restraining influence on him (we had been in close cooperation for eight years) and after he had realized that the regime had irrevocably consolidated its power, he was prepared to compromise his great scientific reputation without scruple. My conviction is that he did this out of conformity and weakness of character, without ever sharing National Socialist convictions. Presumably he was not a party member. But for many years under the Nazi regime he was leader of the 'German Chemical Society' and head of the German chemical delegations to the International Congress in Rome (1939) and on other occasions. ... I am convinced that he is now, after a total reversal of fortune, serious in his efforts to cooperate with American authorities and willing to help alleviate the terrible atrocities committed by the Nazi regime. Presumably, he still justifies his earlier activities with the excuse that in this way he saved some scientific values and prevented worse crimes. But I do not share this view, which is held by numerous German scholars today. [According to Ebbinghaus/Roth (FN 5, p. 48), Kuhn justified his many political functions as protective measures to prevent worse]. The scientific achievement of Richard Kuhn is outstanding and of great importance. I strongly advocate that his scientific work remain unhindered and that he, together with his collaborators, be allowed to continue research for the benefit of science and industry. However, he should no longer be allowed to represent German chemistry in a leading position and should no longer be entrusted with the education of university students. I think that my view is shared by many colleagues in this country who know the work and personality of Professor Kuhn."

In Akademie der Wissenschaften in Heidelberg they worked on dismissing the Jewish or "non-Aryan" scientists. Thus, the then "Reich and Prussian Minister for Science, Education and National Formation" wrote:

> *"I intend to decide in principle the question of the dismissal of non-Aryans among the full and associate members of the Academy of Sciences."*

So, finally, paragraph 5 of the regulations of the Heidelberg Academy also stated: *"Full members can only be those who are German citizens of the Reich (in the Aryan sense) and who have their residence in Heidelberg."* Thus, the latter also ensured that emigrated members who had fled could no longer be part of the Heidelberg Academy of Sciences. Some reactions of the Jewish employees, who were basically forced to resign in the sense of the mentioned paragraph, have been preserved for us archivally: Heinrich Liebmann wrote in handwriting (Fig. 23): *"I hereby declare my resignation from the Heidelberg Academy."* Professor of Roman and Civil Law Fritz Pringsheim wrote (Fig. 24): *"I am a Jew and of Jewish descent. I have no other expression to give. I must leave it*

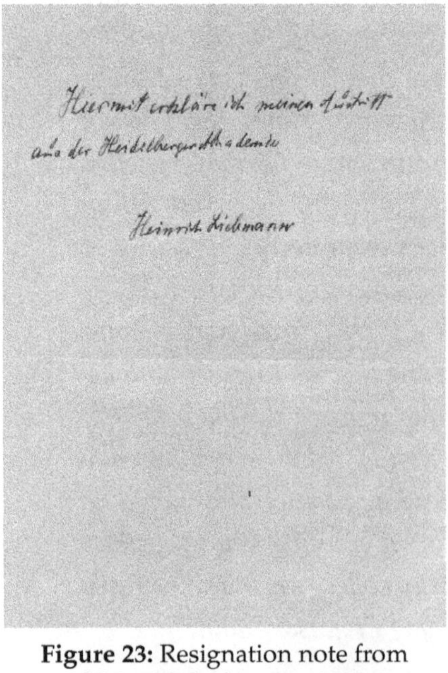

Hiermit erkläre ich meinen Austritt
aus der Heidelberger Akademie

Heinrich Liebmann

Figure 23: Resignation note from Heinrich Liebmann, 1938

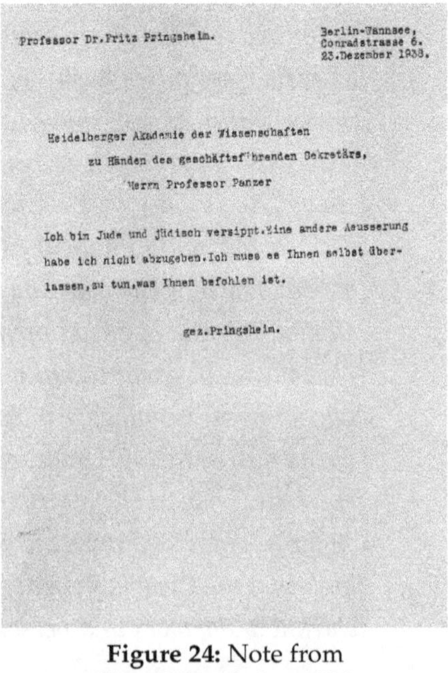

Professor Dr. Fritz Pringsheim.

Berlin-Wannsee,
Conradstrasse 6.
23. Dezember 1938.

Heidelberger Akademie der Wissenschaften
zu Händen des geschäftsführenden Sekretärs,
Herrn Professor Panzer

Ich bin Jude und jüdisch versippt. Eine andere Aeusserung habe ich nicht abzugeben. Ich muss es Ihnen selbst überlassen, zu tun, was Ihnen befohlen ist.

gez. Pringsheim.

Figure 24: Note from Fritz Pringsheim, 1938

to you to do for yourself what you are commanded to do." Georg Bredig, who was working on catalysts in Karlsruhe wrote (Fig. 25): *"If you think it right to remove me as a Jew of German nationality from the list of your members, I leave it to you to do what is necessary."*

Prof. Johann Daniel Achelis (1898-1963), then executive secretary of the Heidelberg Academy of Sciences and director of the Physiological Institute, tried with great commitment to dismiss the Jewish members of the Academy. Some of his letters are preserved in the Heidelberg University Archives. For example, a letter dated February 19, 1937, to "Herr Reichs- und Preußischer Minister für Wissenschaft, Erziehung und Volksbildung Berlin" (Fig. 26) states: *"As the Ministry is aware through repeated reports, considerable difficulties exist at the Heidelberg Academy of Sciences for the regular continuation of its work in that a larger number of members have declared themselves unable to attend meetings as long as Jewish members are full members of the Academy. [...]. The Academy asks the Minister to settle the matters presented, since it hardly seems possible for the Academy to fulfill its tasks in the National Socialist state if Jews belong to it as decision-making members within the meaning of the Reich Citizenship Law."* This request was finally granted, and so

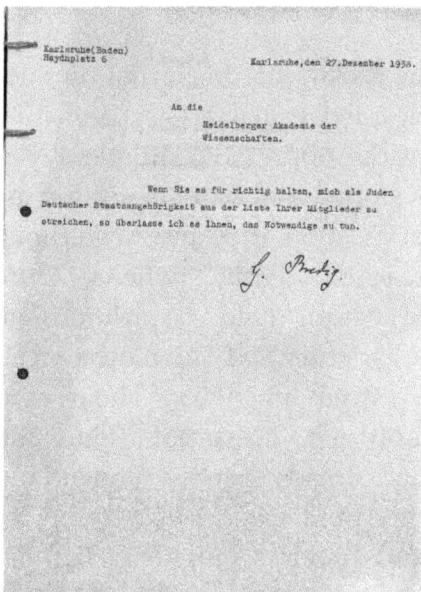

Figure 25: Note from Georg Bredig, 1938

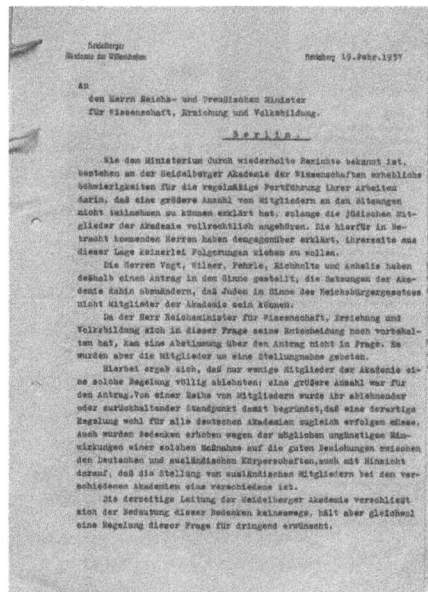

Figure 26: Letter from Professor Johann Daniel Achelis (1898-1963), 1937

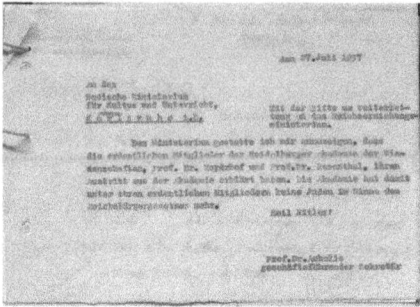

Figure 27: Letter from Professor Achelis, 1937

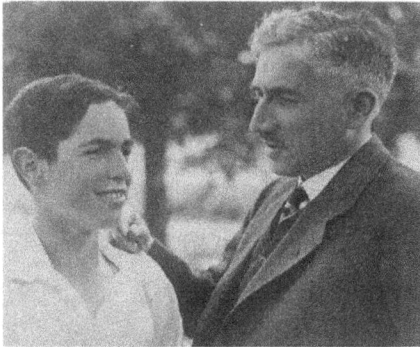

Figure 28: Otto Meyerhof and his son Gottfried in Heidelberg.

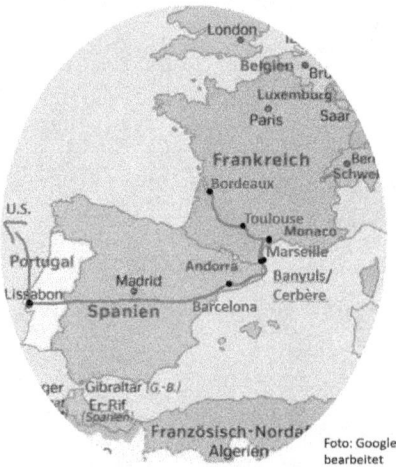

Figure 29: Route of the Meyerhof's escape to America

Achelis wrote on July 27, 1937, a few months after his application (Fig. 27): *"I take the liberty of informing the Ministry that the full members of the Heidelberg Academy of Sciences, Prof. Dr. Meyerhof and Prof. Dr. Rosenthal, have declared their resignation from the Academy. The Academy thus no longer has among its full members any Jew within the meaning of the Reich Citizenship Law. Heil Hitler!"* After the Jewish geologist Salomon Calvi had resigned from the Academy, a colleague of Calvi wrote to Achelis: *"Dear Mr. Achelis, best thanks for your message about the Academy. Now you have a clean room, and I wish you full success in the work of building it up."*

In 1938, the Meyerhof family decided to leave Germany due to the oppressive situation. Via a stopover in Basel disguised as a vacation trip, the Meyerhofs reached Paris, where Otto Meyerhof held a position as a scientist at a biochemical institute in 1938. Their son Gottfried Meyerhof (Fig. 28) had already reached England by this time via a *Kindertransport*, and their daughter Bettina Meyerhof moved from Paris to Swarthmore College in

Philadelphia. After further stays in Toulouse, Bordeaux and Marseille, the Meyerhof couple crossed the border to Spain in 1940 (Fig. 29). They were helped by Varian Fry, a journalist and founder of the Emergency Rescue Committee (Fig. 30), who also brought Heinrich Mann and his wife, Franz Werfel and Alma Werfel, and the Chagall couple across the border. The son Walter Meyerhof was arrested in Banyuls and later helped other Jewish refugees to cross the border there. Hedwig and Otto Meyerhof finally boarded the "Exichorda" in October 1940 and arrived in New York a few days later.

While still on the ship, Otto Meyerhof wrote to the former director of the Rockefeller Foundation, Dr. Lambert (Fig. 31): *"Therefore I write you, for saying, that I would accept any scientific position in U.S.A., which would allow me to get a non-quota visa and to live on a modest scale with my wife and my youngest son."* Otto Meyerhof eventually got a professorship in biochemistry at the University of Pennsylvania (Fig. 32) and six years later was already in possession of a green card (Fig. 33). When the

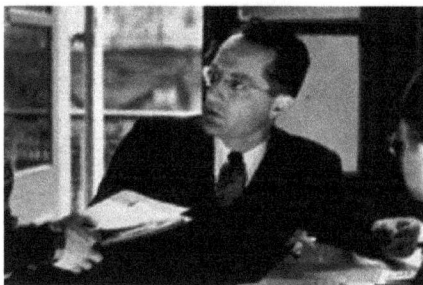

Figure 30: Varian Fry, founder of the 'Emergency Rescue Committee'

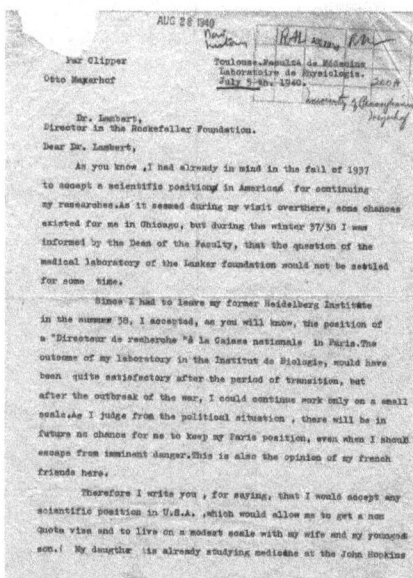

Figure 31: Letter from Otto Meyerhof to Dr Lambert, 1940.

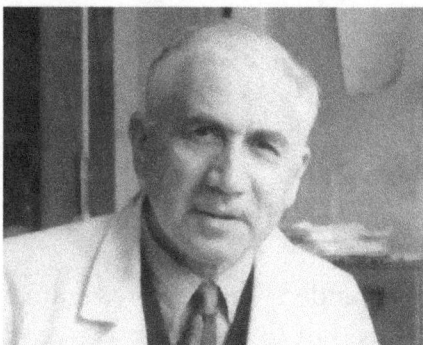

Figure 32: Otto Meyerhof at the University of Pennsylvania

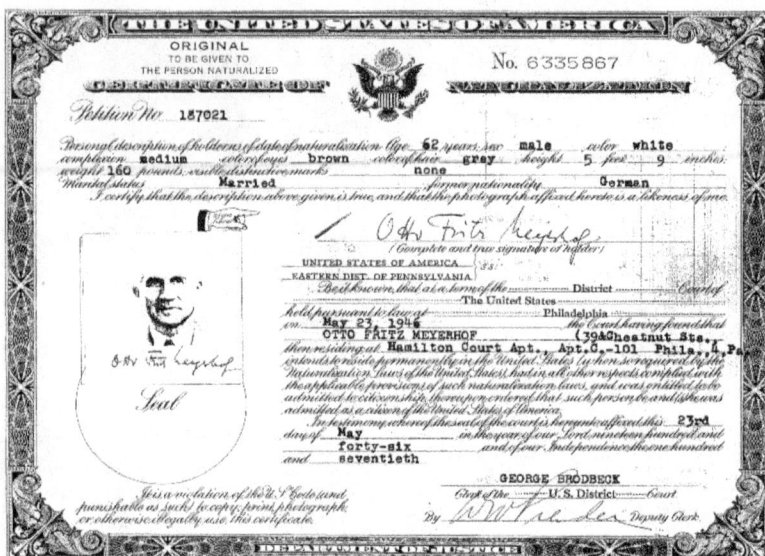

Figure 33: Otto Meyerhof's U.S. 'Green Card'

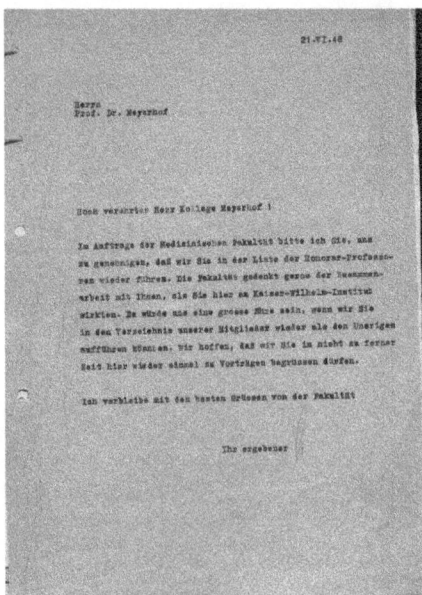

Figure 34: Letter from Dean Hoepke of the University of Heidelberg to Otto Meyerhof, 1948

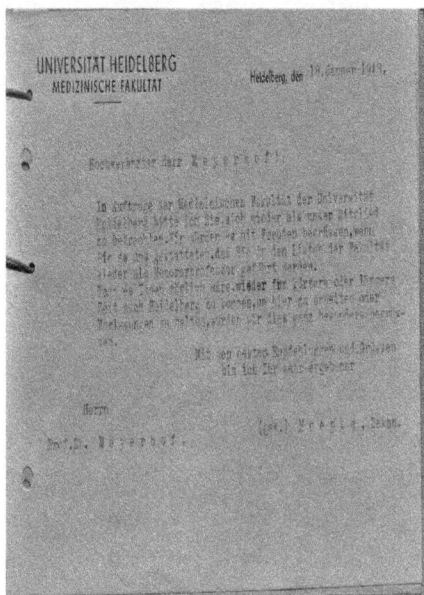

Figure 35: Letter from the University of Heidelberg to Otto Meyerhof, 1948

war ended, there were again requests from Heidelberg for Otto Meyerhof to return to the academy. Thus, the then Dean Hoepke wrote in January 1948 (Fig. 34): *"Esteemed Mr. Meyerhof! On behalf of*

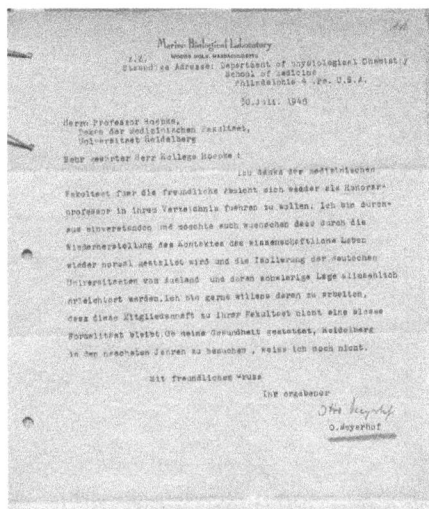

Figure 36: Letter from Otto Meyerhof to Dean Hoepke of the University of Heidelberg

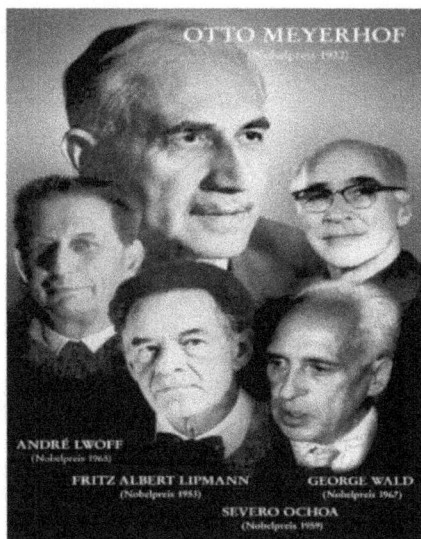

Figure 37: Otto Meyerhof and his four Nobel Prize-winning students

the Medical Faculty of the University of Heidelberg, I ask you to consider yourself again as our member. [...]. If it would be possible for you to come to Heidelberg again for a shorter or longer period of time to work or lecture here, we would particularly welcome it." Further, from the Heidelberg Academy (Fig. 35) it was said: *"It would be a great honor for us if we could again list you as one of our own in the directory of our members."*

Otto Meyerhof responded with the spirit of a great man and scientist who, despite the slights, was able to maintain his optimistic attitude: *"I quite agree and would also like to wish that by restoring contact, scientific life will be restored to normal and the isolation of German universities from abroad and their difficult situation will gradually be alleviated (Fig. 36)."*

Otto Meyerhof lived in the USA until the end and built a new laboratory in Philadelphia. Four of his students also received Nobel Prizes (Fig. 37): Fritz Albert Lipmann (1953), Severo Ochoa (1959), André Lwoff (1965), and George Wald (1967).

In 1951, Otto Meyerhof died in Philadelphia at the age of 67. Richard Kuhn had visited him the very day before. Obviously, there was much to discuss and to debate. Meyerhof's health was already in a delicate state at this time, his cardiological constitution fragile.

David Nachmansohn wrote about Otto Meyerhof:[16] *"As far as his Judaism was concerned, in keeping with his family background, he was completely assimilated. As for many Jews of his generation, his Jewish heritage and the Jewish religion had little meaning for him. Yet he was always conscious of his Jewish ancestry and did not allow himself to be baptized. [...]. But even when the catastrophe of the Hitler era, the persecution of the Jews and the severe suffering that the Nazis inflicted on him and his family, did not change his basic attitude towards the Jewish problem. He regarded this outbreak of anti-Semitism as a throwback to the Middle Ages, an evil force that would disappear with the progress of human society. Then, after the war, when the unimaginably terrible events of the Holocaust became known, it was a horrible shock for him. [...]. His attitude towards Israel was by no means indifferent. He admired the great achievements of the Jews in building a homeland in the desert and also supported Weizmann's efforts to create a scientific center."*

Otto Meyerhof, who throughout his life was concerned not only with philosophy and archaeology, but also with the history of literature and art, and was a great lover of Goethe wrote poetry himself and dedicated an Easter! poem to his wife Hedwig:

"We learned God, and that He created us,
to fulfill the holy work of interpretation,
That He gave us the only profession
To reveal His mystery in wonder.
Was it granted to me, even a thread only
Clear to see on the hem of his mantle,
So remains a breath of my earthly trace
Scattered indissolubly in the starry space.
And all the love we gave each other
In hours full of fear, in happiness and longing
Was sunk into the depths of the universe
And shines before God, like an angel's tears."

---

[16] Nachmansohn D. Die große Ära der Wissenschaft in Deutschland 1900 bis 1933. WVG, 1988. 287

Chapter Two

Otto Meyerhof:
Pioneer of Modern Biochemistry

Walter Nickel

Otto Meyerhof was one of the world's most important scientists of the 20th century. He discovered "the gear train of chemical cycles in the degradation of food substances and the associated energetic coupling for the universal storage of chemical binding energy in the form of adenosine triphosphate (ATP), the direct _operating material_ for the various work performances of all living beings," as Hans-Hermann Weber, his first scientific collaborator, put it. The impact of his scientific work on the research of subsequent generations was tremendous. His discoveries are not only documented in all the biochemistry textbooks of our time, but also form the basis for today's biomedical research in many respects. The alteration of carbohydrate metabolism in tumor cells and the resulting therapeutic approaches are a good example of this. The discoveries of Otto Meyerhof and their impact on today's research can be summed up in the words of Thomas Kuhn: "There was a biochemistry before Meyerhof and one since."

The chemical basis of energy metabolism in the context of the work performance of living organisms.

The groundbreaking scientific discoveries of Otto Meyerhof in the first half of the 20th century revealed fundamental aspects of the energy metabolism of living organisms that still form the basis of modern biochemistry. He was one of the first to pose the question of how living organisms can harness energy released from the oxidation-mediated breakdown of food substances for work performance. He was among the pioneers of the life sciences who applied the laws of physics to cellular systems in order to decipher the energy metabolism of living organisms on the basis of the principles of thermodynamics. In this context, he chose an experimental model system that allowed him to precisely quantify a work output of a biological system under controlled conditions, the muscle isolated in intact form. In doing so, he used sophisticated instruments, some of which he had developed himself, that allowed him to determine muscle activity generated by electrical stimuli, for example, in terms of stroke height and the frequency of muscle twitches. These experiments could also be carried out in a controlled manner with regard to the availability of oxygen. In addition, Otto Meyerhof and his co-workers succeeded in isolating and quantifying defined intermediates of metabolism under various experimental conditions. Under the title "The Chemical Processes in Muscle and their Relation to Work Output and Heat Generation", Otto Meyerhof summarized his early work, most of which he had carried out single-handedly during his time in Kiel, and which was awarded the Nobel Prize in Medicine in 1922 (Fig. 1).

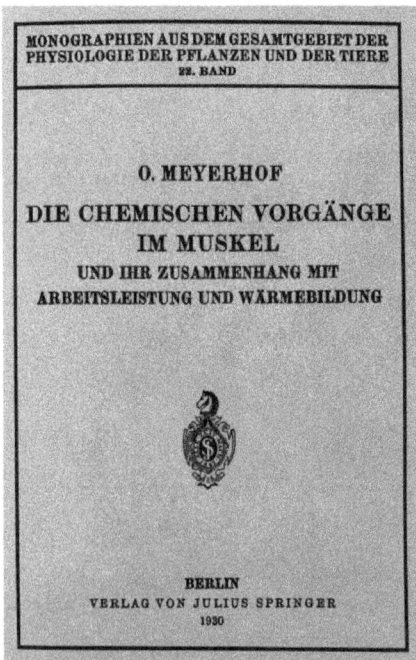

Fig. 1: Otto Meyerhof (1930) "The chemical processes in muscle and their connection with work performance and heat generation".

A fundamental question to which Otto Meyerhof devoted himself during his time in Kiel concerned the function of lactic acid formation in active muscle. It was already known at that time that lactic acid is formed and accumulates in the course of the utilization of carbohydrates from glucose during heavy exercise of the muscle tissue, but the reason for this was completely unknown. Through his systematic studies of the chemical processes during the three principal states of the muscle, the resting state, the activity phase and the recovery phase, Otto Meyerhof was able to demonstrate that the lactic acid formed during the activity phase disappears again during the recovery phase. The underlying mechanisms and their meaning, however, initially remained mysterious to the scientific world at that time. It was Otto Meyerhof who, by means of his experimental and theoretical approaches, first recognized that the lactic acid is not completely oxidized to carbon dioxide and water during the muscle's recovery phase. Instead, he was able to demonstrate that lactic acid is converted back into glucose via pyruvate in the course of a process we now call gluconeogenesis. Even more, the glucose is converted to its storage form, glycogen, during the muscle's recovery phase. This process consumes energy, which is provided by the portion of lactic acid that is oxidized to carbon dioxide and water via pyruvate during the recovery phase. Otto Meyerhof recognized these relationships and developed from them the original form of the famous Meyerhof quotient, which relates the amount of lactic acid that is converted back into glycogen to the amount of lactic acid that is completely oxidized for energy production (Fig. 2).

Beyond its specific importance for deciphering the chemical processes in active muscle tissue, this discovery had a fundamental significance for the recognition of biochemical principles of metabolism. Otto Meyerhof had discovered the first biochemical metabolic cycle (Fig. 3).

Many others were to follow, such as the citrate and urea cycles. Otto Meyerhof had discovered a basic principle and thus laid the foundation of modern biochemistry.

Meyerhof Quotient:

$$\frac{\text{Zu Glykogen resynthetisierte Milchsäure}}{\text{Zur Energiegewinnung oxidierte Milchsäure}}$$

Fig. 2: The Meyerhof quotient in its original form (1922).

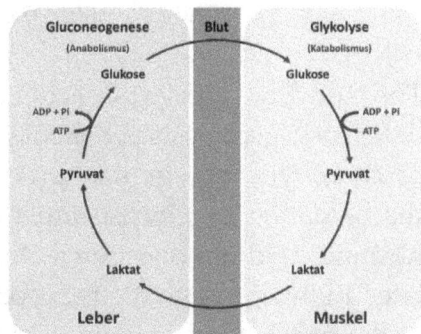

Fig. 3: The cycle of glycolysis and gluconeogenesis during muscle activity and recovery discovered by Otto Meyerhof, which revealed a basic principle of biochemistry.

However, Otto Meyerhof's Nobel Prize-winning research revealed other basic principles as the central foundations of biochemistry. In an extended form of the Meyerhof quotient, Otto Meyerhof's pioneering experimental approaches elucidated the relationship between oxygen uptake and lactic acid formation in terms of a fixed stoichiometry. With his later contributions to the identification of the reactions and their catalyzing enzymes of glycolysis, the conversion of glucose to pyruvate, Otto Meyerhof also provided a contribution to the deciphering of the function of lactic acid formation (Fig. 4).

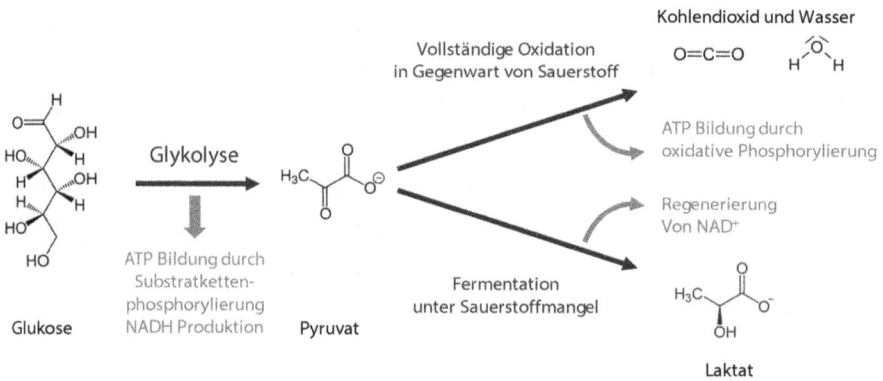

Fig. 4: The two principal mechanisms for the synthesis of ATP in biological systems: Substrate chain phosphorylation in glycolysis and oxidative phosphorylation in mitochondria. In the presence of oxygen, pyruvate is completely oxidized to carbon dioxide and water. In the absence of oxygen, the reduction equivalents (NADH) formed in glycolysis are converted back to NAD+ by the conversion of pyruvate to lactate, so that ATP can be continuously produced in glycolysis under these conditions.

The function of lactic acid formation is that under oxygen deficiency, glycolysis is the sole source of energy in the breakdown of carbohydrates. In this process, the electrons released during the oxidation of glucose must be transferred to an acceptor, the nicotinic acid amide dinucleotide (NAD+), which was discovered later. In this process, the reduced form of NAD+ is formed, NADH. In the presence of oxygen, NADH can be used in the course of the respiratory chain localized in the mitochondria by the transfer of electrons from NADH to oxygen with the formation of water via intermediate energy storage in the form of a proton gradient at the inner mitochondrial membrane for the intermediate storage of chemical binding energy in the form of adenosine triphosphate (ATP). This process is referred to as oxidative phosphorylation. A second form of ATP formation is substrate chain phosphorylation, mentioned above and shown in Fig. 4, in which the oxidation of glucose in energy-producing partial reactions of glycolysis is coupled to the formation of ATP. The structure-function relationships and molecular mechanism underlying reversible energy storage through the formation of ATP were later elucidated by Karl Lohmann and Otto Meyerhof during their time together in Berlin and Heidelberg in the 1920s and 1930s.

In the absence of oxygen, substrate chain phosphorylation is the only way to form ATP because oxidative phosphorylation requires oxygen to form ATP in mitochondria. However, in the absence of oxygen, glycolysis can only continuously supply ATP via substrate chain phosphorylation if NAD+ can be regenerated from the NADH formed during the glycolysis process. This necessity is met by converting the end product of glycolysis, pyruvate, into lactic acid in a redox reaction (Fig. 4).

The electrons released from NADH in this reaction are transferred to pyruvate, regenerating NAD+. By this biochemical trick, NAD+ is recovered from NADH so that the conversion of glucose via pyruvate to lactic acid can proceed continuously to form ATP via substrate chain phosphorylation (Fig. 5).

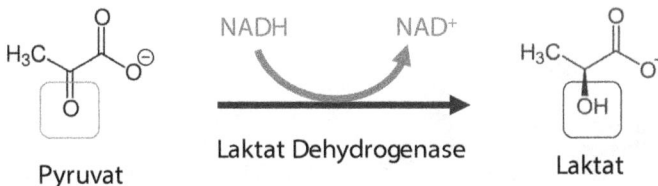

Fig. 5: The formation of lactic acid (lactate) from pyruvate. This is a redox reaction in which the oxidized form of NADH, NAD+, is regenerated. The electrons released in this process are transferred to the carbonyl group (C=O; green box) of pyruvate, which is thereby reduced to an alcohol (-OH; blue box).

The ATP formed by this metabolic mechanism in the absence of oxygen can enable muscle activity in the absence of oxygen, although oxidative phosphorylation to form ATP in mitochondria is not possible under these conditions (Fig. 6).

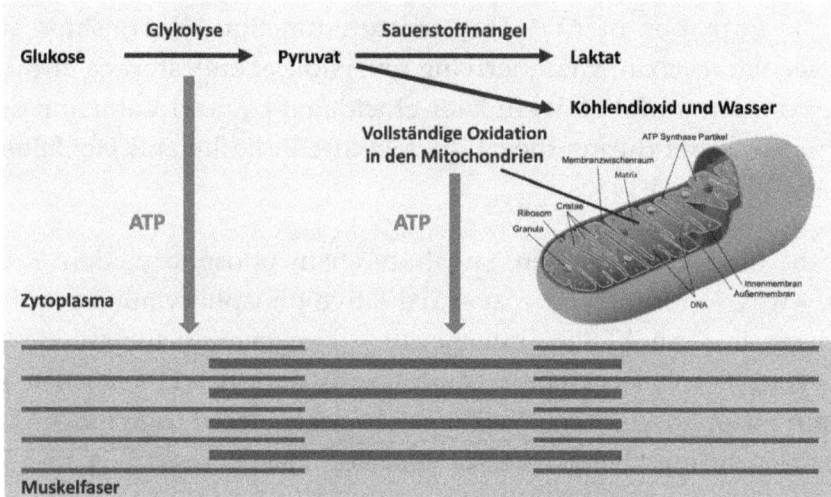

Fig. 6: Schematic representation of ATP sources for muscle contraction under aerobic and anaerobic conditions.

In later work, Otto Meyerhof was able to describe another mechanism that allows muscle under oxygen deficiency to generate ATP independently of glycolysis for muscle work. Together with Einar Lundsgaard, David Nachmansohn and Karl Lohmann, he deciphered the function of creatine phosphate (Fig. 7).

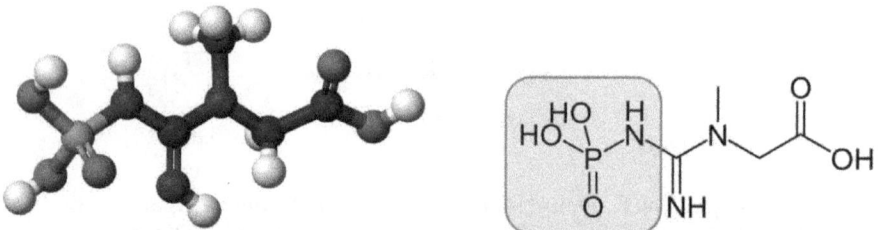

Fig. 7: Structure of creatine phosphate.

This is also a high-energy, phosphate-containing compound with a similar group transfer potential compared to ATP. In fact, the high-energy adenosine triphosphate can be generated by transferring the phosphate group from creatine phosphate to adenosine diphosphate to form creatine (Fig. 8).

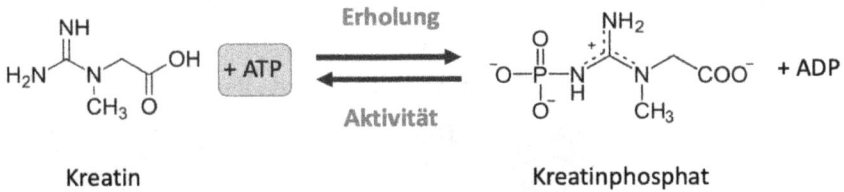

Fig. 8: Reversible conversion of creatine phosphate and ADP to creatine and ATP during muscle activity by phosphate group transfer.

The stoichiometry of creatine phosphate and ATP in muscle is about 5:1, so that in this way ATP can be regenerated to a significant extent independently of the oxidation of carbohydrates for muscle contraction. Modern spectroscopic techniques can be used to determine the concentrations of creatine phosphate, adenosine triphosphate, and the phosphate cleaved from them in the three phases of muscle activity. Here, the formation of inorganic phosphate (Pi) reveals that ATP is cleaved during the activity phase. However, the total amount of ATP does not change. Instead, creatine phosphate is consumed, thereby keeping the amount of ATP constant. In the recovery phase, creatine phosphate is recycled. The ATP amount remains constant in all described phases of muscle activity.

These relationships were recognized early on by Otto Meyerhof and his colleagues and form the basis of our current understanding of the energy metabolism of muscle work. In addition, Otto Meyerhof and his colleagues discovered one of the first examples of group transfer reactions catalyzed by enzymes (transferases), for which numerous other examples were later identified.

Deciphering the structure and function of adenosine triphosphate (ATP), the direct "fuel" of all living things.

The crucial question, the solution of which Otto Meyerhof and Karl Lohmann succeeded in solving during their time together, first in the 1920s in Berlin and later in the 1930s at the Kaiser Wilhelm Institute for Medical Research (today's Max Planck Institute for Medical Research) in Heidelberg (Fig. 9), and which brought them the greatest fame, was the question, completely unsolved at that time, of how the energy obtained during the oxidation of food substances could be reversibly stored temporarily and mobilized in a controlled manner for work activities such as muscle activity.

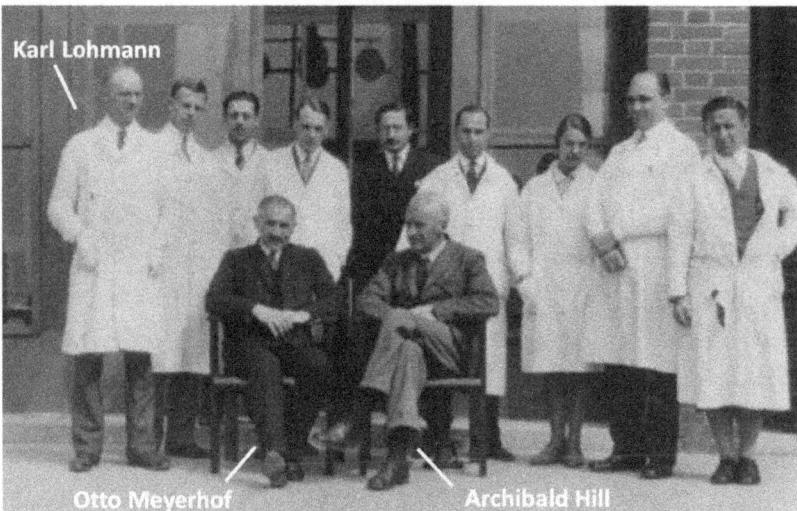

Fig. 9: Otto Meyerhof with Karl Lohmann, Archibald Hill and his colleagues in front of the then Kaiser Wilhelm Institute for Medical Research in Heidelberg (Photo: MPI for Medical Research, Heidelberg).

It was already clear to Otto Meyerhof at this time that it would be extremely unlikely that the energy released during the oxidation of food substances would be directly linked to energy-consuming processes such as muscle work. Instead, it seemed much more plausible to him that these processes were decoupled in time. The fundamental question to be solved, therefore, was how the chemical binding energy contained, for example, in carbohydrates such as glucose and released during their oxidation (catabolism) could be reversibly conserved in energy-rich molecules so that it could be used, if needed, for energy-consuming processes (anabolism) at a later time. This puzzle was solved through the close collaboration of the analytical chemist Karl Lohmann and the physiologically minded biochemist Otto Meyerhof, who possessed outstanding skills both in the strategic planning and execution of experiments and in their interpretation on the basis of the laws of thermodynamics.

Karl Lohmann succeeded already in Berlin in the isolation and structural elucidation of ATP, which he was able to isolate from the active muscle and identify in its chemical structure (Fig. 10).

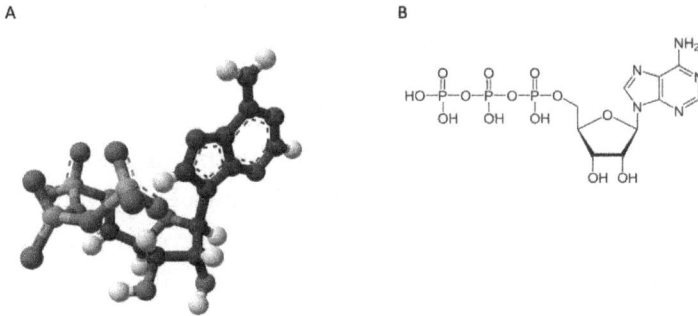

Fig. 10: Structure of adenosine triphosphate.

A.) Spatial molecular model of ATP based on X-ray structural analysis by Olga Kennard, N. W. Isaacs, W. D. S. Motherwell, J. C. Coppola, D. L. Wampler, A. C. Larson, D. G. Watson (1971). "The Crystal and Molecular Structure of Adenosine Triphosphate. "Proceedings of the Royal Society of London. Series A, Mathematical and Physical Sciences 325: 401-436. DOI:10.1098/rspa.1971.0177).

B.) Chemical structural formula of ATP

Here he decomposed ATP into its components adenine, ribose and three phosphate groups using boiling hydrochloric acid and identified these components by analytical chemical methods. He identified the phosphate groups from ATP, for example, by the formation of colored molybdenum complexes. These observations were published in the journal "Natural Sciences" with the title *"On the pyrophosphate fraction in muscle"* and are considered in modern biochemistry as the discovery of ATP as the universal source of energy, which all living beings obtain from the oxidation of food substances and which are directly or indirectly coupled to all energy-consuming processes of living beings. However, the isolation of ATP and its structural elucidation did not immediately lead to the recognition of the significance of Karl Lohmann's fundamental discovery. Only close collaboration with Otto Meyerhof revealed the secret of ATP, the reversible storage of chemical binding energy in the anhydride bonds linking the phosphate groups of the ATP molecule. Ultimately, Meyerhof and Lohmann demonstrated that hydrolysis of the outer anhydride bond leads to the formation of ADP and inorganic phosphate, and that the energy released in this process enables muscle contraction. Since ATP and creatine phosphate are interconvertible, muscle contraction by the creatine phosphate buffer can even occur over a period of time independently of the ongoing ATP production of glycolysis. In retrospect, the discovery of the structure and function of ATP is considered on a par with the discovery of the structure and function of DNA, the genetic material of all living things, in terms of its importance to biology and medicine. The award of the Nobel Prize to Karl Lohmann and the award of a second Nobel Prize to Otto Meyerhof would have been justified without any doubt.

Otto Meyerhof was one of the beacons of the life sciences in the 20th century. Together with a few other scientists, such as Otto Warburg, he was one of the decisive pioneers of modern biochemistry, which he decisively shaped as a new and independent scientific discipline from the field of physiological chemistry. In his time, he was one of the first to systematically investigate the energy metabolism of biological systems on the basis of the laws of physics, especially the principles of thermodynamics. Hans-Herrmann Weber, his first academic collaborator in Berlin in the 1920s, summed up Otto Meyerhof's epoch-making scientific discoveries and achievements in one sentence by saying, "Otto Meyerhof discovered the gear train of chemical cycles in the breakdown of food substances and the associated energetic coupling for the universal storage of chemical binding energy in the form of adenosine triphosphate (ATP), the direct operating material of all living things." It has the principles of chemical processes in the various states of the muscle, the function of lactic acid formation and its relationship to oxygen uptake, the first biochemical cycle with the reconversion of lactic acid via glucose into glycogen, a substantial part of the intermediates and enzymes of glycolysis, discovered and deciphered the structure and function of creatine and arginine phosphate (together with Karl Lohmann and other former students and collaborators) and, to a certain extent as the crowning achievement of his incomparable scientific discoveries, the structure and function of adenosine triphosphate as the link between energy-supplying and energy-consuming metabolic processes. How could one form a comprehensive picture of the biochemical processes in biological systems today without knowledge of the energy-rich organic phosphate compounds such as ATP? Thus, Thomas Kuhns logically states, "There is a biology and medicine before and one since Meyerhof." Moreover, Otto Meyerhof was not only one of the decisive pioneers of modern biochemistry, with his groundbreaking discoveries he also laid the foundations for the biomedical research of the present day. The manipulation of carbohydrate metabolism by tumor cells and the resulting therapeutic and diagnostic approaches are a good example of this.

Beyond his scientific achievements, Otto Meyerhof also distinguished himself as a friend, mentor, and collaborator. He shared lifelong friendships with both Otto Warburg and Archibald Hill. He encouraged his students and gave them great freedom so that they could develop into outstanding, independent scientists. Thus encouraged by Otto Meyerhof, four of his former students (Fritz A. Lipmann in 1953, Severo Ochoa in 1959, André Lwoff in 1965, and George Wald in 1967; Fig. 11) later received the Nobel Prize themselves. The outstanding scientific achievements of these scientists were undoubtedly fostered by the scientific culture shaped by Otto Meyerhof.

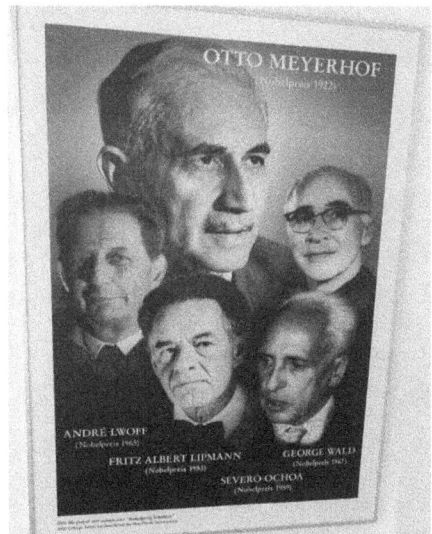

Fig. 11: Otto Meyerhof and his students, who were later themselves awarded the Nobel Prize (photo collage MPI for Medical Research, Heidelberg; individual images from the archive of the Max Planck Society).

In particular, his close friendly relationship with Archibald Hill testified to an open scientific exchange in the otherwise difficult political relations in Europe after the First World War. In his Nobel Prize speech, he expressed the great pleasure he took in receiving the joint award from a British and a German scientist, which they accepted in Stockholm in 1922. All the more depressing is the persecution and injustice of expulsion that befell Otto Meyerhof, his family and the Jewish community as a whole during the Nazi era. None of the family members who remained in Europe during this time survived the Holocaust.

Lecture as part of the Ruperto Carola Lecture Series 2021 at Heidelberg University: "Otto Meyerhof - a life as a scientist between fame and expulsion".

https://www.uni-heidelberg.de/de/transfer/kommunikation/ruperto-carola-ringvorlesung

https://www.youtube.com/watch?v=Uep2bcTRVqk

Selected literature

Hans-Hermann Weber – Otto Meyerhof: Die Umsetzung der Energie der Nahrungsstoffe in die Leistungen der Lebewesen

Eberhard Hofmann – Otto Meyerhof – Humanist und Naturforscher Von der Philosophie zum Nobelpreis

Eberhard Hofmann – Otto Meyerhof und Karl Lohmann – Wegbereiter der heutigen Biochemie im Schatten ihrer Zeit

Eberhard Hofmann – Otto Meyerhof and the Exploration of Glycolysis – Outstanding Research in an Inhumane Era

Eberhard Hofmann – Otto Warburg und Otto Meyerhof – die Geschichte einer Freundschaft

Maren Emmerich – Cells Flexing Their Muscles

Heiner Schirmer und Stephan Gromer – Meyerhof in Heidelberg: Der Aufbruch der Zellbiologie

Otto Meyerhof – Die chemischen Vorgänge im Muskel und ihr Zusammenhang mit Arbeitsleistung und Wärmebildung

Otto Meyerhof – Energy Conversions in Muscles (Nobel Lecture, Dec 12, 1923)

Chapter Three

Anti-Semitism at Heidelberg University 1933 - 1945

Frank Engehausen

"The end of the war found Heidelberg University ... outwardly intact, inwardly it had been almost completely destroyed by the twelve years of dictatorship," it says at the end of the chapter on the "Third Reich" in Eike Wolgast's history of Heidelberg University.[1] A large part of the internal destruction was due to anti-Semitism, which also broke out at the universities in 1933 and clearly demonstrated that the principles of the academic culture formed in the 19th century no longer counted for anything under National Socialism. At the 550th anniversary of Heidelberg University in 1936, Reich Minister of Education Bernhard Rust openly admitted this in his speech, justifying the racially motivated purges of previous years: There was no longer any place at the university for all those "who do not belong to us by blood and nature, and who therefore lack the ability to shape science out of the German spirit": a lack of preconditions and freedom from values were no longer its essential characteristics; "science as a system" was only possible "on the basis of a living", i.e. National Socialist, worldview.[2]

The means by which those whose "blood and nature" were not conducive to the National Socialist type of university were ousted from the Ruperto-Carola, who bore responsibility for this, and how those affected reacted to the injustice perpetrated against them will be outlined in the following. The focus will be on the first years of the dictatorship, and the later phase will only be looked at insofar as

---

[1] Eike Wolgast, Die Universität Heidelberg 1386-1986, Berlin u. a. 1986, S. 167.

[2] Das nationalsozialistische Deutschland und die Wissenschaft, Heidelberger Reden von Reichsminister Rust und Prof. Ernst Krieck, Hamburg 1936, S. 19.

dismissed Heidelberg professors and their relatives were affected by the anti-Semitic measures of the war years. It is not possible in this format to explore all facets of anti-Semitism at Heidelberg University from the beginning to the end of the "Third Reich"; in particular, the question of the extent to which anti-Semitism found expression in academic teaching is left out. The prehistory of anti-Semitism at Heidelberg University can also only be roughly sketched.

Prehistory

Anti-Semitism did not come upon the University of Heidelberg in 1933 like an unforeseeable natural phenomenon, but had already made itself felt beforehand. It was - which may seem paradoxical only at first glance - a concomitant of the comparatively early emancipation of Jews in Baden and the comparatively liberal appointment practice at Heidelberg University, which did not reserve its professorships for members of Christian denominations. As early as 1861, Gustav Weil, a Jew, had been appointed to a Heidelberg chair, and by 1914 a total of 60 professors had taught at the Ruperto Carola who were Jews or, from an anti-Semitic racist point of view, were regarded as such because their ancestors had been Jews.[3] Resentment against Jewish professors probably also existed in Heidelberg during this period; however, there were no widespread conflicts, such as those that emerged in 1879 in the Berlin anti-Semitism dispute.

This changed after World War I, when two members of the Heidelberg faculty became conspicuous as anti-Semites: In 1920, at the request of the Heidelberg Philosophy Faculty, the Baden Ministry of Culture withdrew the teaching license of Arnold Ruge, a private lecturer in philosophy, after he had massively attacked the university's Jewish professors at an event organized by the Deutschvölkischer Schutz- und Trutzbund. More serious than the Ruge case was the case of

---

[3] Vgl. dazu z. B. die Ausstellung der Universitätsbibliothek Heidelberg „Juden an der Universität Heidelberg. Dokumente aus sieben Jahrzehnten", die 2002 in Heidelberg und in Jerusalem gezeigt wurde: http://www.alemannia-judaica.de/ images/Images%20460/Heidelberg%20juden_hd%20Dokumente.pdf.

Philipp Lenard in 1922, since
he was not one of the marginal
figures on the teaching staff, but
a Grand Ordinary: Nobel Prize
winner for physics and director
of the University Institute of
Physics, which he refused to
close or flag down on the day of
the funeral of the assassinated
Foreign Minister Walter
Rathenau, since in his opinion
students were not allowed to
"laze around because of a dead
Jew." Lenard thus provoked
the storming of his institute by
socialist students and workers;

Fig. 1: Philipp Lenard (1862-1947)

disciplinary proceedings conducted against him by the university
in 1923 ended with the mild sanction of a reprimand - the political
eccentric was allowed to get away with this aberration in view of his
great scientific reputation.[4]

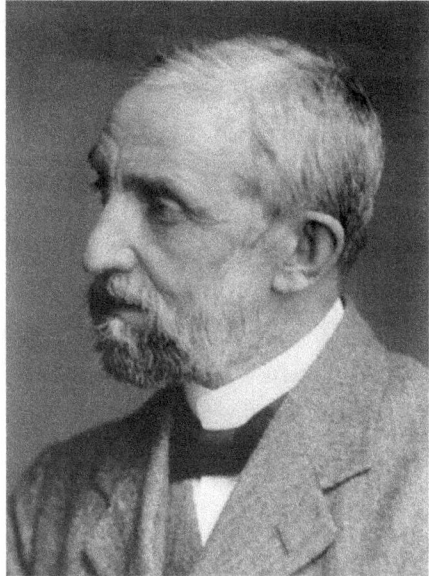

The third incident was different, the protracted dispute over the
private lecturer and later associate professor of statistics Emil
Julius Gumbel: After two anti-Semites had caused scandals among
the teaching staff with Ruge and Lenard, this time it was a Social
Democrat, pacifist and Jew who attracted disciplinary proceedings
because his provocative statements about the war challenged
the basic consensus on national values. While the disciplinary
proceedings petered out after the first incident in 1924, also because
of intervention by the Ministry of Education, the conflict escalated
in 1932 to the revocation of his teaching license.[5] Even though for the
professors involved in Gumbel's dismissal, his political statements

---

[4] Vgl. Marie-Thérèse Roux, Die Universität Heidelberg und der „Fall Philipp Lenard".
Der Umgang mit der antirepublikanischen Provokation eines Hochschullehrers
1922/23, in: Heidelberg. Jahrbuch zur Geschichte der Stadt 25 (2021), S. 97-120.

[5] Vgl. Christian Jansen, Emil Julius Gumbel. Portrait eines Zivilisten,
Heidelberg 1991, S. 30-40.

were the decisive judging factors, the case became an anti-Semitic éclat due to the involvement of National Socialist students. They had collected signatures against the disfavored Jewish professor and staged the "Gumbel case" retrospectively as a local prelude to the national revolution of 1933. In general, it can be stated that anti-Semitic attitudes at Heidelberg University were widespread in student circles during the years of the Weimar Republic. Nearly one-third of the students belonged to corporations that admitted only "German students of Aryan descent," and by the 1930 AStA elections, the National Socialist Student League had already become the strongest faction, holding more than one-third of the seats.

Dismissals in 1933

Wherever the legal equality of Jews had led to integration successes, anti-Semitism appeared all the more sharply in 1933 to reverse this development. For Heidelberg University, this meant that it came vehemently to the fore after the National Socialist takeover. Its omnipresence was thus primarily the result of measures acting from outside and not of an internal process of disintegration, even though anti-Semitism had already spread before 1933. It reached its breakthrough barely four weeks after the National Socialist takeover in Baden and the replacement of the top positions in the university's supervisory authority, the Ministry of Culture in Karlsruhe, which was henceforth led by the Nazi party journalist Otto Wacker. Wacker assigned the leadership of the university department in the ministry to a member of the Heidelberg university faculty, Associate Professor of Classics Eugen Fehrle, who had also held a teaching position in folklore since 1926, had joined the NSDAP in 1931, and had been appointed by the Gauleiter in 1932 as the party's "university advisor at the University of Heidelberg."[6] In his new position, Fehrle was quickly promoted to ministerial councilor, and in the office he held until 1936, he played a central role in the university's staff

---

[6] Vgl. Frank Engehausen, Das badische Ministerium des Kultus und Unterrichts, in: Ders., Sylvia Paletschek u. Wolfram Pyta (Hg.), Die badischen und württembergischen Landesministerien in der Zeit des Nationalsozialismus, Stuttgart 2019, S. 321f.

harmonization. So, if some contemporaries sought to convey the impression that anti-Semitism was something entirely alien to the university, this was not entirely true, for one of Heidelberg's professors, though an outsider by status, subject, and political orientation, played a significant role in opening the floodgates to it.

On April 5, 1933, the provisional government of Baden issued a decree according to which all "members of the Jewish race"

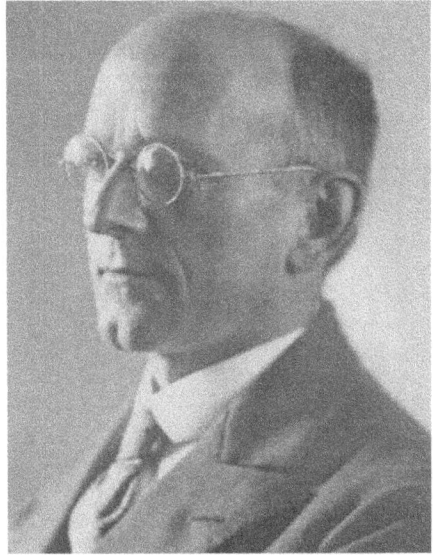

Fig. 2: Eugen Fehrle (1880-1957)

employed in the public service were to be granted leave of absence - according to the pseudo-biological definition, one was considered such if at least one of the grandparents was "non-Aryan". Just as the University of Heidelberg was beginning to implement the leaves of absence, the Reich Law on the Restoration of the German Race came into force on April 7. It was both harsher and milder than the Baden decree it repealed: harsher in that non-Aryan members of the civil service were dismissed and not just given leave of absence, milder in that there were exemption clauses that benefited non-Aryans who had entered the civil service before 1914, even as soldiers fighting in World War I or who had lost their fathers or sons there.[7]

How to deal with the discrepancies between the Baden decree and the Reich law was initially unclear in many places, and at the University of Heidelberg the practice of granting leave of absence continued until the end of April, which could have very distressing consequences in individual cases: The terminally ill honorary professor of mineralogy Victor Goldschmidt, for example, had his letter of leave of absence forwarded

---

[7] Vgl. ebd., S. 332-343.

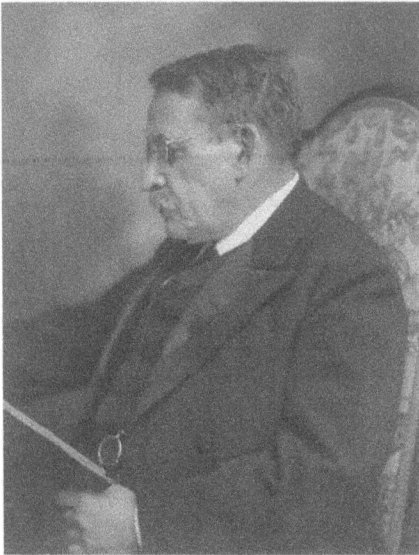

Fig. 3: Victor Goldschmidt (1853-1933)

to a Salzburg sanatorium, where he died in early May 1933 with the impression that he had been expelled from the university, even though he fell under the exemption clauses of the Reich Law.[8]

The university committees reacted differently to the first anti-Semitic measures of the National Socialist regime. Immediately on April 5, when the Baden decree on leave of absence became known, the Medical Faculty agreed to record concerns about the decree in a memorandum to be sent to the Ministry of Culture, which was signed by Dean Richard Siebeck. In this memorandum it was emphasized "that German Jewry participates in great achievements in science and that great medical personalities have emerged from it. Especially as physicians we feel obliged to represent the standpoint of true humanity within all the requirements of the people and the state and to assert our concerns where there is a danger that responsible attitudes will be displaced by purely emotional or instinctive forces and that the great German task will suffer as a result. We must insist that the legal consciousness be preserved and that the position of the professional civil service be protected.[9] The Faculty of Natural Sciences and Mathematics took a similar view and supported a statement by the university against the anti-Semitic measures. The Faculty of Philosophy and the Faculty of Law were more reserved, and the Senate of the University could not bring itself to an open protest on April 10. Although they drafted a resolution pointing out that the "compulsory leave of absence of colleagues for whose employment the university

---

[8] Vgl. Frank Engehausen, Die Josefine und Eduard von Portheim-Stiftung für Wissenschaft und Kunst 1919-1955. Heidelberger Mäzenatentum im Schatten des dritten Reiches, Heidelberg u. a. 2008, S. 83f.

[9] Universitätsarchiv Heidelberg B 3026/4a.

itself bears joint responsibility" was contrary to their sense of justice and that the leaves of absence would cause considerable damage to the university,[10] to all appearances this resolution remained a draft and was not sent to Karlsruhe.

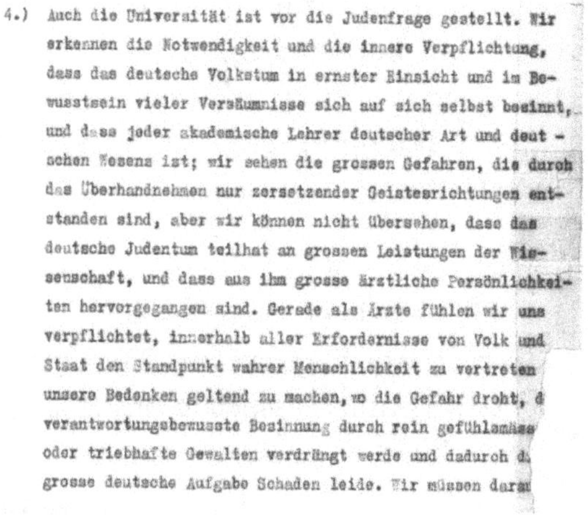

4.) Auch die Universität ist vor die Judenfrage gestellt. Wir
erkennen die Notwendigkeit und die innere Verpflichtung,
dass das deutsche Volkstum in ernster Einsicht und im Be-
wusstsein vieler Versäumnisse sich auf sich selbst besinnt,
und dass jeder akademische Lehrer deutscher Art und deut -
schen Wesens ist; wir sehen die grossen Gefahren, die durch
das Überhandnehmen nur zersetzender Geistesrichtungen ent-
standen sind, aber wir können nicht übersehen, dass das
deutsche Judentum teilhat an grossen Leistungen der Wissenschaft, und dass aus ihm grosse ärztliche Persönlichkei-
ten hervorgegangen sind. Gerade als Ärzte fühlen wir uns
verpflichtet, innerhalb aller Erfordernisse von Volk und
Staat den Standpunkt wahrer Menschlichkeit zu vertreten
unsere Bedenken geltend zu machen, wo die Gefahr droht, d
verantwortungsbewusste Besinnung durch rein gefühlsmäss
oder triebhafte Gewalten verdrängt werde und dadurch d
grosse deutsche Aufgabe Schaden leide. Wir müssen dara

Fig. 4: From the memorandum of the Medical Faculty of April 5, 1933.

The confidence of the university bodies in the weight of their own voice was obviously not very great, and instead of open protest, they resorted to a tactic of evasion and stalling, as well as interceding on behalf of individual affected persons, for whom they tried to obtain exemptions. However, these efforts largely came to naught, giving the impression that the university administration had silently allowed the arbitrariness to pass. One of those affected, the botanist Gerta von Ubisch, recorded the following in her memoirs: "One wondered how it was possible that the universities did not vote against these laws, that they did not unanimously stand up for their colleagues. If all the university professors, doctors, lawyers had done so, if they had all gone on strike, the laws could never have been carried out. There are a number of reasons why they did not. At one point, the timing of the legislation was very clever. During the Easter vacations, when a great many lecturers who had not been warned were away, a vote was

---

[10] Ebd. Vgl. dazu auch Birgit Vezina, „Die Gleichschaltung" der Universität Heidelberg im Zuge der nationalsozialistischen Machtergreifung, Heidelberg 1982, S. 35f.

taken by the rest who were in favor of the regime or yet indifferent to it, and those who returned were faced with a fait accompli. Secondly, the law with the restrictions demanded by Hindenburg did not affect very many full professors at all, since almost all of them had been in one or another position in the war or had been recruited for vital tasks in the hinterland, in the stage: it thus affected almost only younger professors who had not participated in the war. Given the caste distinction and the sharp boundary that exists at German universities between full professors and non-professors, the former were thus not very interested in the latter."[11]

That von Ubisch has drawn the lines of conflict here only a little sharper than they may actually have been becomes apparent when one looks at the numbers. Among those dismissed in 1933 for racist reasons were four full professors or scheduled associate professors, three honorary professors, three non-scheduled professors, and six private lecturers:[12]

The academic establishment was thus actually less affected than those lecturers who had not yet gained a firm foothold. Six other members of the Heidelberg faculty who had been declared non-Aryan renounced their office and teaching authorization, although they fell under the exemption clauses, signaling that they no longer saw any professional prospects at the university in light of the spreading anti-Semitism. How the protective efforts of the university administration in favor of individuals failed in the process is shown by the case of the ancient historian Eugen Täubler, who did not want to make use of the rector's offer to suspend his leave of absence in consideration of his war service, but instead applied for a semester off in order to prepare his departure from Heidelberg. To remain in office as a mere "tolerated person" did not seem bearable to Täubler, and he also turned down the supposedly honorable departure that the university wanted to give him by transferring him to retirement.[13]

---

[11] Zwischen allen Welten. Die Lebenserinnerungen der ersten Heidelberger Professorin Gerta von Ubisch, hg. v. Susan Richter u. Armin Schlechter, Ostfildern 2011, S. 91.

[12] Vgl. die Zahlen in Wolgast, Universität (wie Anm. 1), S. 144.

[13] Vgl. Dorothee Mussgnug, Die vertriebenen Heidelberger Dozenten. Zur Geschichte der Ruprecht-Karls-Universität nach 1933, Heidelberg 1988, S. 54-57.

The main responsibility for bureaucratic anti-Semitism on the part of the university was borne by the rector and the deans of the faculties - two of them took office extra-rotationally in April 1933, because the incumbents elected six months earlier, by then labeled non-Aryan, resigned, although as participants in the war they fell under the exemption clauses of the Law for the Restoration of Professional Civil Service: the mathematician Arthur Rosenthal and the jurist Ernst Levy. From the latter, the law deanship was taken over by Wilhelm Groh, who, by joining the SA, quickly sided with the National Socialists, who until then had been very weakly represented on the Heidelberg faculty. Thus, the key figure in the racist dismissals of 1933 was not a party man, but the historian Willy Andreas, who had been elected rector in the fall of 1932 and was an old-established national-liberal-conservative full professor, who also later did not join the NSDAP and was probably not anti-Semitic in his personal views. Nor can he be accused of having a weak political backbone in general: In the last days of his rectorate in September 1933, he found critical words in a private letter to the Baden Minister of Culture on the elimination of academic autonomy through the introduction of the so-called Führer principle at the universities;[14] however, the anti-Semitic legislation of spring 1933 obviously did not have such a fundamental significance for him that he would have decided to protest clearly.

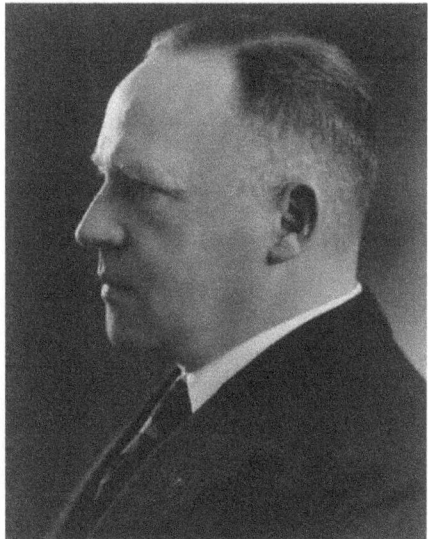

Fig. 5: Willy Andreas (1884-1967)

---

[14] Vgl. Volker Sellin, Die Rektorate Andreas, Groh und Krieck 1933-1938, in: W. U. Eckart, V. Sellin u. E. Wolgast (Hg.), Die Universität Heidelberg im Nationalsozialismus, Heidelberg 2006, S. 12f.; Vezina, Gleichschaltung (wie Anm. 19), S. 74-77.

At least Andreas made efforts in several cases to find individually tolerable solutions, although this was made more difficult by the fact that anti-Semitic agitators from the university itself stabbed him in the back several times during negotiations with the Ministry of Culture. An example of this is the case of Gerta von Ubisch, who offered several options for interpretation, since for her, as a non-tenured lecturer, the law applied only mutatis mutandis. In addition to Andreas, the war historian and later Heidelberg rector Paul Schmitthenner, who had defected to the National Socialists, also supported her, seeing her non-Aryan origins as compensated for by Prussian aristocratic blood. The mineralogist Hans Himmel and the physician Johannes Stein, representing the non-ordained, assessed the case quite differently. They informed in a letter to the Ministry of Culture "that Mrs. von Ubisch is to be regarded unambiguously as a Jewess, descent on her mother's side. It therefore seems to us unjust and out of place to spare her, especially since in her case there are probably no special scientific achievements as perhaps in the case of Prof. Meyerhof, and opinions are also very divided about her teaching ability."[15]

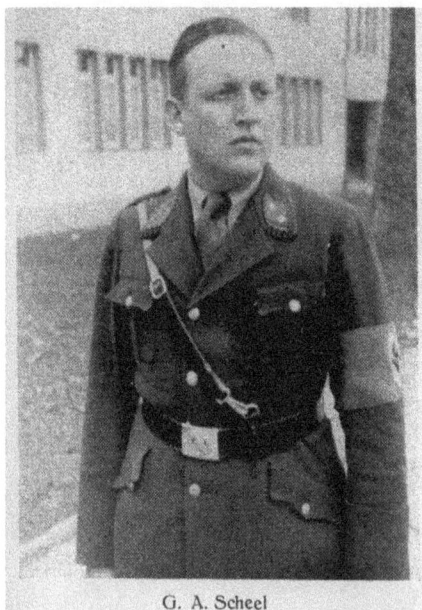

G. A. Scheel

Fig. 6: Gustav Adolf Scheel (1907-1979)

Himmel and Stein found support in this matter from the student leader Gustav Adolf Scheel, who had considerable influence in the first phase, because he was able to fill the vacuum of the hardly existing old party comrades of the NSDAP at the Ruperto-Carola with his good contacts to the Gau leadership of the party.

How the bureaucratic anti-Semitism of 1933 at Heidelberg University was perceived from

---

[15] Generallandesarchiv Karlsruhe 235 5007, Schreiben von Hans Himmel an den Hochschulreferenten Eugen Fehrle vom 27.8.1933.

the outside is difficult to assess. When Andreas resigned from the office of rector in the fall of 1933, articles appeared in the bourgeois Heidelberg daily press praising his balancing conduct in office - and thus also his efforts to mitigate the fate of individual non-Aryan professors. The local Nazi press reacted to this with sharp counter-articles criticizing Andreas as a representative of a vanished era of liberal science who had tried to delay the national awakening at the university. Quite bluntly, the racist purges at the university were commented on abroad, for example, in an anonymous letter to Rector Andreas from Zurich in September 1933, the author of which asked him, on behalf of several dozen Jewish Americans, "whether it is right for you to keep the money begged by Israelites to rebuild your university. After they behave as Huns and barbarians and act deceitfully and meanly towards your German colleagues, they may still have so much honor as pork lard sandwich eaters to return this money for the victims of barbarism i.e. refugees".[16]

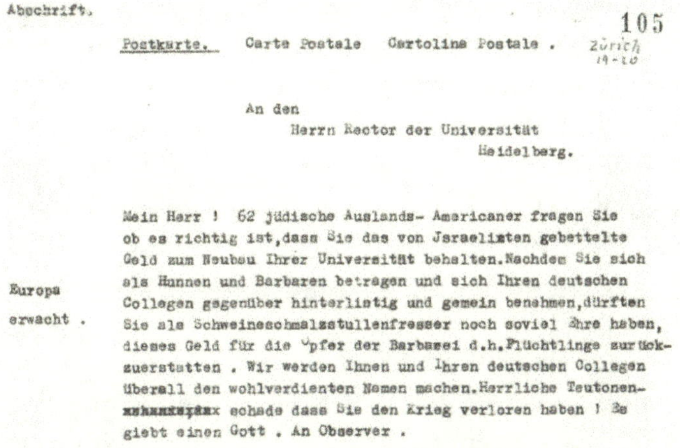

Abschrift.

Postkarte.   Carte Postale   Cartolina Postale .   Zürich
                                                       19-10

105

An den
    Herrn Rector der Universität
                        Heidelberg.

Europa
erwacht .

Mein Herr ! 62 jüdische Auslands- Amerikaner fragen Sie
ob es richtig ist,dass Sie das von Israeliten gebettelte
Geld zum Neubau Ihrer Universität behalten.Nachdem Sie sich
als Hunnen und Barbaren betragen und sich Ihren deutschen
Collegen gegenüber hinterlistig und gemein benehmen,dürften
Sie als Schweineschmalzstullenfresser noch soviel Ehre haben,
dieses Geld für die Opfer der Barbarei d.h.Flüchtlinge zurück-
zuerstatten . Wir werden Ihnen und Ihren deutschen Collegen
überall den wohlverdienten Namen machen.Herrliche Teutonen-
xxhxxxxyxxx schade dass Sie den Krieg verloren haben ! Es
giebt einen Gott . An Observer .

Fig. 7: Anonymous letter from Zurich to the Rectorate, September 1933.

[16] Universitätsarchiv Heidelberg B 1015/4b.

Students and student body

While the rector, senate and deans acted reactively in 1933 and tried to achieve an at least partially lenient interpretation of the anti-Semitic measures, the National Socialist students took the offensive soon after the seizure of power in March 1933. A key role in this was played by the student leader Scheel, who used his good party-political contacts to ensure that a general enrollment ban on Jewish students was issued for the Baden universities as early as April 13, 1933. Like the Baden decree on leave of absence, this ban also proved to be a hasty measure, as the regulations under Reich law were less rigorous. The "Law against Overcrowding in German Schools and Universities" of late April 1933, in fact, only stipulated a *numerus clausus* for non-Aryan students. Their share of total students was not allowed to exceed five percent, and the upper limit for new enrollments was 1.5 percent. More important than this racist numerus clausus, however, was the everyday discrimination against Jewish students. In addition, the general anti-Semitic legislation reduced their chances of finding access to an academic profession to a minimum - a major incentive to study was thus removed. This can be clearly seen in the number of students: In the summer semester of 1933, 177 students classified as non-Aryan were enrolled in Heidelberg, more than half of them in the Medical Faculty. Already in the following semester, there were 76, far less than half, and in 1937 only five Jews were still studying in Heidelberg.[17]

Little is known about the fates of the non-Aryan students, most of whom left the university without a degree. In the majority of cases, it is likely to have been a matter of frustrated withdrawal rather than active ousting. There are, however, examples of the latter, such as the case of philology student Heinz Stern, who was denounced by a bookseller in July 1933 for a statement about the Reichstag fire, sentenced by a special court to a one-year prison term, and denounced in the National Socialist press as a "Judenlümmel" with a "flippant mouth." After his release from prison, Stern was punished

---

[17] Vgl. Eike Wolgast, Die Studierenden, in: Eckart, Sellin u. Wolgast, Universität (wie Anm. 14), S. 62f.

with relegation by the university's disciplinary court in July 1934 because of this incident.[18]

That verbal discrimination was the order of the day and that fisticuffs against non-Aryan students also occurred can be assumed, but cannot be substantiated in detail in the sources. Orchestrated anti-Semitic riots, as the National Socialist students had used in the past, occurred only sporadically in 1933, for example at the beginning of the summer semester with the occupation of the house of the Jewish fraternity Bavaria by SA students. Bavaria, like the second Jewish fraternity based in Heidelberg, Ivrea, was forced to disband by the Baden Ministry of Culture right in the summer semester of 1933. Instead of the Jews, the National Socialist students directed their activities in 1933 mainly at the actually or supposedly communist students. Thus, in June 1933, the Heidelberg student newspaper and also the local party newspaper published a list with the names of 26 students of both sexes who were to be removed from the university because they had "demonstrably espoused communism" - emphasizing that "an extraordinarily large percentage of these people are Jews."[19] The publication of such a blacklist was not enough, however, as the National Socialist activists had to realize: the bureaucratic implementation of the relegations dragged on for months, and from then on the student leadership around Scheel tried to better coordinate their advances with the relevant committees. On the whole, provocations among fellow students remained on a small scale, for example, at the end of April 1933 with the decree of the student body president that "Jewish and Marxist students were no longer allowed to enter the refectory" until a swastika flag that had allegedly been stolen there was retrieved.[20]

The targets of the National Socialist students' actions were not primarily their unpopular fellow students, but the professors who had been sidelined for political or racist reasons. Here, too,

---

[18] Vgl. Universitätsarchiv Heidelberg StudA Heinz Stern; Der Führer vom 30.7.1933.

[19] Vgl. Der Heidelberger Student vom 1.6.1933.

[20] Zit. nach: Arno Weckbecker, Die Judenverfolgung in Heidelberg 1933-1945, Heidelberg 1985, S. 170.

the thrust was primarily political, as when SA students dragged the dentist Georg Joseph Blessing out of his lecture and took him into "protective custody" because he was accused of financial irregularities.[21] But non-Aryan professors were also affected by provocative actions: The private practice of dermatologist Siegfried Bettmann, for example, was strikingly boycotted in the course of the general "Jewish Action" on April 1, 1933; on the same day, his son Hans-Walter, who had been informed that he was to lose his position as assessor at the district court, committed suicide.[22] Although this action may have been directed against the Jewish doctor and not against the university professor, Bettmann, like his fated colleagues who were initially allowed to remain in office due to the exemption clauses of the Purge Law, was affected by the lecture boycott that the National Socialist students issued against the non-Aryan lecturers who remained in 1933 without consulting the university committees.

Like this lecture boycott, the book burning that took place in Heidelberg on the University Square on May 17, 1933, was a genuine initiative of the National Socialist students. On posters and in the press, the student body, the district leadership of the NSDAP, and the Heidelberg branch of the Kampfbund für deutsche Kultur called for the public burning of "antivölkisch propaganda writings and Jewish-Marxist decomposition literature," with the request going out to every student to thoroughly sift through their own book collections. The books of which authors were burned in Heidelberg have not been handed down. Of the non-Aryan Heidelberg authors, only Gumbel, who had already been dismissed the previous year, was apparently affected; at least Scheel, as a speaker at the book burning, mentioned his name alongside those of other alleged "criminals against the German spirit."[23] Unlike in other university cities, no member of the academic faculty was among the speakers at the book burning. One does not necessarily have to see a conscious distancing of the professors from this event; perhaps Scheel just wanted the stage reserved entirely for

---

[21] Vgl. Mussgnug, Dozenten (wie Anm. 13), S. 50f.

[22] Vgl. ebd., S. 63f.

[23] Der Heidelberger Student vom 1.6.1933.

the students. In a certain sense, the book burning in mid-May 1933 marked the conclusion of symbolic political anti-Semitic actions by the National Socialist student body, which Scheel shortly thereafter called upon, not for moderation, but for discipline. By virtue of his office as leader of the Heidelberg student body, he henceforth forbade any individual political action by students at Heidelberg University. Violators were threatened with immediate expulsion from the party.

Dismissals 1935-1940

A good year and a half passed before coordinated anti-Semitic actions by the student body resumed, during which the non-Aryan professors who remained at the university due to the exemption clauses tried to come to terms with the oppressive conditions for them and, above all, had to deal with their marginalization in university life, which was accelerated quite a bit in 1934 by withdrawing their examination authorization. An impetus for further measures was provided in January 1935 by the Law on the Dismissal and Transfer of University Teachers, which gave universities the means to reprofile faculties. The Baden Ministry of Culture planned this for the Heidelberg Law Faculty, among others, which was to be converted into a so-called Stoßtrupp Faculty, i.e., a model National Socialist faculty, but this seemed impossible as long as full professorships were held by non-Aryans. Thus, with the approval of the university administration, attempts began to get rid of those concerned, including Walter Jellinek, by transferring them to other German universities, by relieving them of their official duties, or by retiring them.

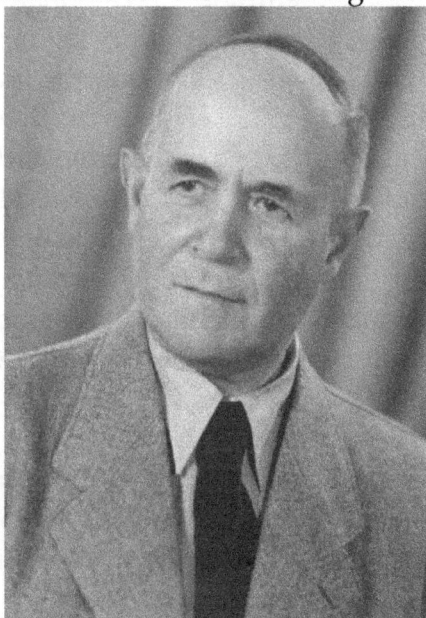

Fig. 8: Walter Jellinek (1885-1955)

These attempts were flanked by intensified boycott actions by the student body: In the Faculty of Natural Sciences, for example, it organized actions against Arthur Rosenthal, whom the Baden Ministry of Culture wanted to have transferred out of the country, since two non-Aryan mathematicians were unacceptable for the faculty in the long run. In May 1935, the student council organized parallel lectures and exercises given by assistants, and when Rosenthal complained about this to the rector, the latter

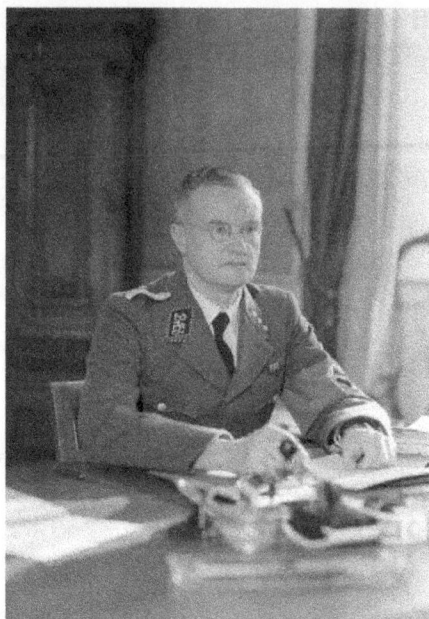

Fig. 9: Wilhelm Groh (1890-1964)

declared that he would intervene against breaches of order, but that he could not oppose the efforts of the National Socialist German Student League - this would be incompatible with his own "National Socialist attitude."[24] The man who thus denied his colleague protection from arbitrary action by the National Socialist students was Andreas's successor: the lawyer Wilhelm Groh, in office since the fall of 1933, who was the first rector after the introduction of the Führer principle at the universities to come to office not by election but by political appointment. He differed from his predecessor in that he had demonstratively defected to the National Socialist camp by joining the SA in 1933; what he had in common with him was the endeavor to intervene, at least cautiously in individual cases, in a mitigating manner in favor of non-Aryan professors. In the face of political pressure, however, Groh tended to buckle quickly, which was also related to the fact that he was only the nominal "leader" of the university and had to come to terms in everyday life with a "leadership staff" that framed him politically and included, among others, the student leader Scheel.[25]

---

[24] Zit. nach: Mussgnug, Dozenten (wie Anm. 13), S. 71.

[25] Vgl. Paul Christopher Leo, Wilhelm Groh – Erster Rektor der Ruperto-Carola in der NS-Zeit, Hamburg 2012

The tough and, for those affected, degrading struggle to oust individual non-Aryan professors from their positions at the university finally ended with the "Nuremberg Race Laws" and the implementing decrees issued in their wake in the fall of 1935. Since the non-Aryans were now no longer German citizens, they could no longer be civil servants and were to be retired - this applied analogously to honorary professors as well as to non-civil servant associate professors and private lecturers. The racial purges thus carried out in Heidelberg were even more

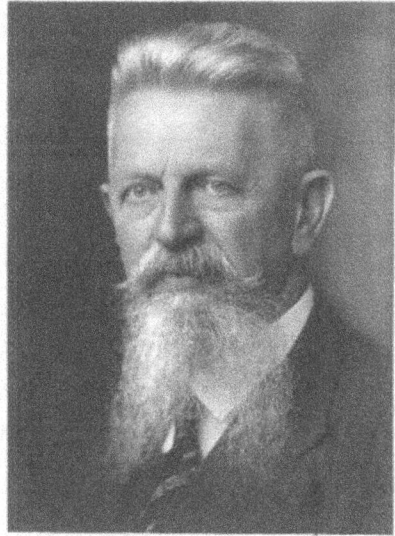

Fig. 10: Wilhelm Salomon-Calvi (1868-1941)

extensive than the dismissals of 1933. As far as the status groups were concerned, the ratio was reversed in 1935: A dozen full professors, scheduled associate professors and honorary professors, and nine non-scheduled professors and private lecturers were affected.[26] Among them were a number of scientific luminaries, including Otto Meyerhof, to whom this lecture series is dedicated, and the geologist and honorary Heidelberg citizen Wilhelm Salomon-Calvi, whose teaching license was revoked after he emigrated to Turkey. He had accepted a call to Ankara - with a heavy heart, as he noted in a letter to the Ministry of Culture in Karlsruhe, and in an effort to "work culturally for our fatherland in Ankara and, as far as it is in my power, to do honor to the German name".[27]

---

[26] Vgl. die Zahlen in Wolgast, Universität (wie Anm. 1), S. 145.

[27] Zit. nach: Mussgnug, Dozenten (wie Anm. 13), S. 74.

Two years after this wave of dismissals, bureaucratic anti-Semitism raged again: it was given fresh impetus by the entry into force of the German Civil Service Law at the beginning of 1937, according to which not only civil servants had to possess the characteristics of a citizen of the Reich, but also their spouses had to be of "German or kindred blood" - "non-Aryans of affinity", as the word monstrosity used to designate this state of affairs, were consequently to be retired. Exceptions could only be granted

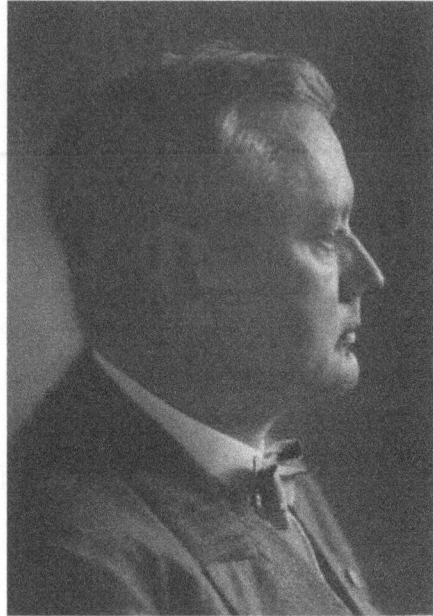

Fig. 11: Ernst Krieck (1882-1947)

by the Reich Minister of the Interior or the "Deputy of the Fuehrer" - for this to happen, the university administration, the Baden Ministry of Education, the Reich Ministry of Education, and also party offices would have had to pull together, which, however, was not the case with any of the Heidelberg professors concerned. On the contrary, in several cases the university administration pushed for the removal of non-Aryan people from the teaching staff: the art historian August Grisebach had long been suspected of political unreliability, and his chair had aroused requests for reassignment, since the war historian Paul Schmitthenner was finally to be given a full professorship, so that Grisebach's dismissal in 1937 was virtually overdue. In the case of the Egyptologist Hermann Ranke, the university prepared the dismissal in 1937 with disciplinary proceedings for favoring a deserter, and also in the case of the classical philologist Otto Regenbogen, disciplinary proceedings preceded the retirement: he had named his wife as "Aryan" in a questionnaire because he had not known until then that one of her grandmothers had only been baptized as a child.[28]   Such pseudo-biological nonsense had not

---

[28] Vgl. ebd, S. 96-103.

been questioned for a long time - especially not by the rector Ernst Krieck, who had advanced academically with an NSDAP party card and had also only reached the top of the university because of his political merits.[29]

However, even under Krieck's rectorship, the university leaders were not guided by blind anti-Semitic zeal throughout, but continued to strive for partial mitigations: This happened, for example, in the case of the full honorary professor and lecturer Eberhard von Künssberg, who was the scientific director of the German Legal Dictionary and only taught part-time at the university. The law faculty wanted to keep him in office for reasons of prestige, which succeeded with Krieck's intercession to the Reich Ministry of Education.[30] Krieck was less successful in his efforts on behalf of his philosophical colleague Karl Jaspers, whose dismissal was urged by the Baden Ministry of Education because he was married to a so-called Volljüdin. Krieck advocated an early emeritus status for Jaspers instead of his retirement, arguing that Jaspers "would have had to ask for emeritus status in the foreseeable future anyway" because of his failing health; also, the dismissal of such a renowned philosopher would cause an unwelcome stir. Krieck, however, did not succeed with this in the Reich Ministry of Education; Jaspers was retired.[31]

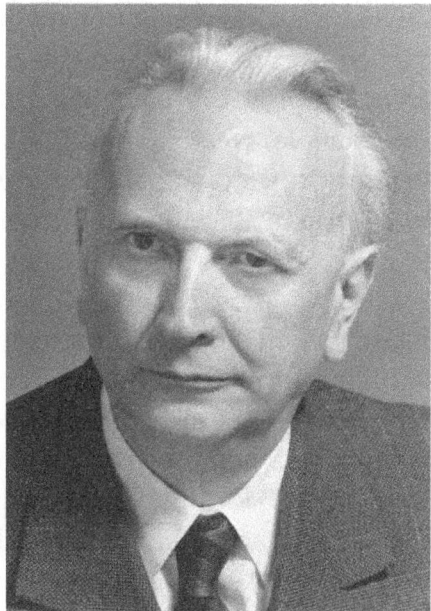

Fig. 12: Karl Jaspers (1883-1969)

---

[29] Vgl. Vanessa Hilss, Prof. Dr. Ernst Krieck: „Einordnen [...] nach allen Seiten hin. Der NS-Wegbereiter in der Erziehung, in: Wolfgang Proske (Hg.), Täter – Helfer – Trittbrettfahrer. Bd. 7: NS-Belastete aus Nordbaden und Nordschwarzwald, Gerstetten 2017, S. 198-209.

[30] Vgl. Mussgnug, Dozenten (wie Anm. 13), S. 106.

[31] Vgl. ebd., S. 98-100.

Fates of the dismissed professors

It is difficult to generalize about the fate of the non-Aryan and non-Aryan Heidelberg lecturers who were dismissed between 1933 and 1940, since their prospects varied greatly depending on their status, age, professional qualifications and the time of dismissal: As a rule, the dismissed civil servant lecturers were entitled to a pension, which relieved them of at least existential material worries if they had completed a corresponding number of years of service. The situation was quite different for dismissed honorary professors with teaching assignments or private lecturers with grants, who had to reorient themselves without any income. An obvious option was professional self-employment, which, however, could quickly become a mere fiction due to the discriminatory anti-Semitic legislation against doctors or lawyers. Since employment in research and teaching in Germany was practically out of the question, emigration was the way out, chosen by more than half of those affected in Heidelberg. The associate professor of modern German literature Richard Alewyn, for example, went to France after his dismissal in June 1933, held visiting professorships in Paris and London, moved with his family to Austria in 1935, fled to Switzerland in 1938, and was finally able to emigrate to the United States in 1939.[32] Of those affected by the second wave of dismissals, mention should be made of the jurist Ernst Levy, who in 1935 attempted to forestall his retirement by applying for emeritus status. Levy wanted to follow his children, who had already emigrated to the USA, and had to conduct lengthy negotiations with the Baden Ministry of Education and the Reich Ministry of Education about the payment of his emoluments abroad - in the end, he could not avoid the now obligatory Jewish property levy and the Reich flight tax.[33]

The mathematician Arthur Rosenthal, also a victim of the 1935 dismissals, initially remained in Heidelberg after his early retirement, was deported to the Dachau concentration camp for several weeks

---

[32] Vgl. ebd., S. 140.
[33] Vgl. ebd., S. 151.

after the pogrom of November 9, 1938, and only then accelerated his emigration efforts: He went to the Netherlands in July 1939 and to the USA in March 1940; it was not until the end of 1941 that he managed to catch up with his mother, who had been deported to Gurs in the meantime. The latest emigrant among those released from Heidelberg was the ancient historian Eugen Täubler, who had made his living in 1938 as a lecturer at the Berlin Hochschule für die Wissenschaft des Judentums. He emigrated to the USA in March 1941.[34] Not all of those dismissed from Heidelberg managed to escape in time before being deported to concentration camps: Richard Werner, a surgeon and head of the medical department of the Institute for Cancer Research, who was granted leave of absence in 1934, went from Heidelberg to Brno, where he served as clinic director until the so-called Rest of Czechoslovakia was annexed by the Germans in 1939. In 1942 he was deported to Theresienstadt, where he died. The lawyer Leopold Perels was deported from Heidelberg to Gurs and lived to see the end of the war in France. The gynecologist Maximilian Neu, who had run a practice in Heidelberg until the ban on non-Aryan doctors in 1938, escaped the mass deportation of Baden Jews to France in October 1940 by committing suicide. He and his wife took cyanide when a police officer came to pick them up for deportation.[35]

Also threatened with deportation during the war years were the wives of those who remained in Heidelberg and were dismissed as non-Aryan. This was true for Karl Jasper's wife Gertrud and for Katharina, the widow of the lawyer Eberhard von Künssberg, who died in 1941, who had to fear being deported to concentration camps until the last days of the war. After the war, the last Nazi rector of Heidelberg, the war historian Paul Schmitthenner, claimed credit for having made attempts to protect both of them.[36] The fact that, on the one hand, he had no qualms about holding high positions in the dictatorial system

---

[34] Vgl. ebd. S. 166f.

[35] Vgl. ebd., S. 146, 172, 136.

[36] Vgl. Karl Jaspers Korrespondenzen. Politik, Universität, hg. v. Carsten Dutt u. Eike Wolgast, Göttingen 2016, S. 545f., Schreiben von Schmitthenner an Karl Jaspers vom 21.4.1948.

of injustice, and that during his rectorate non-Aryan graduates of the Ruperto Carola were stripped of their doctorates as if on an assembly line, and that, on the other hand, he was concerned about the fate of the Jewish wife of a former faculty colleague, is only an apparent paradox.

Similar behavior can be seen in the case of Eugen Fehrle, who was responsible for the dismissals of non-Aryan lecturers as a ministerial councilor in the Baden Ministry of Culture from 1933 to 1936,

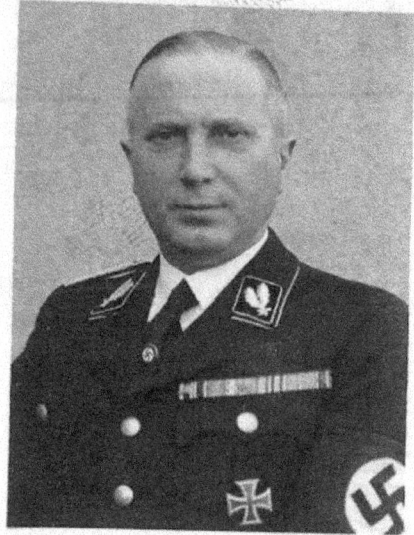

Fig. 13: Paul Schmitthenner (1884-1963)

but who made some effort to have Viktor Goldschmidt's widow removed from a deportation list after his return to Heidelberg as a full professor of folklore and dean in 1942. When this failed, she too committed suicide.[37]

Conclusion

Were men responsible for the anti-Semitism at the University of Heidelberg in the years 1933 - 1945 who were not anti-Semites at all and did not even believe the pseudo-biological nonsense on which the repressive measures were based? This question cannot be answered clearly, since it is beyond the capacity of a historian to reconstruct personal convictions. Only the writings and deeds of the people responsible at the time are accessible for evaluation, and from these an ambivalent picture emerges. Of the persons in leadership positions, i.e. the rectors and the deans, one will probably have to attest to a closeness to anti-Semitism, especially to Ernst Krieck, according to

---

[37] Vgl. Engehausen, Portheim-Stiftung (wie Anm. 8), S. 136-138.

their publications, even though he ultimately threw in the towel with the leading race theorists of the regime because of his völkisch-political anthropology. The fact that they were not ideological propagandists of anti-Semitism did not, however, prevent those responsible in Heidelberg from implementing the repressive measures and thus recognizing the bizarre logic of anti-Semitism. It would be easy to explain this with obedience to the authorities or a lack of civil courage - but in the end it is hardly comprehensible, since all those involved were men who, by taking up the scientific profession, had made rationality their basis of existence, or should have done so.

Even in the case of the agitators among the student body and young scientists who emerged as consistent anti-Semites in 1933, it is no longer possible to prove that they were ideological fanatics. What is undoubted, however, is that they used anti-Semitism as a means to achieve personal goals: in the case of the student leader Scheel, for political profiling,[38] which enabled him to pursue a steep career in the SS, and in the case of Johannes Stein, for advancement to the chair of internal medicine without adequate professional qualifications.[39] The case of the mineralogist Hans Himmel stands out in terms of repugnance of character; he only openly appeared as a National Socialist when his mentor Victor Goldschmidt was dying, and then tried to sabotage the modest efforts of the Heidelberg rectorate to obtain exemptions for individual non-Aryan lecturers by making representations in higher political places.[40] Himmel, however, was not the only one guilty of abandoning intra-institutional solidarity; rather, this reproach can be levelled at all functionaries of Heidelberg University who tolerated the disenfranchisement of their non-Aryan colleagues without contradiction and participated in its administrative execution.

---

[38] Vgl. Philipp T. Haase, Gustav Adolf Scheel. Studentenführer, Gauleiter, Verschwörer. Ein politischer Werdegang, in: Wolfgang Proske (Hg.), Täter – Helfer – Trittbrettfahrer. Bd. 8: NS-Belastete aus dem Norden des heutigen Baden-Württembergs, Gerstetten 2019, S. 295-325.

[39] Vgl. Axel W. Bauer, Innere Medizin, Neurologie und Dermatologie, in: Eckart, Sellin u. Wolgast, Universität (wie Anm. 14), S. 720-728.

[40] Vgl. Engehausen, Portheim-Stiftung (wie Anm. 8), S. 98f.

Chapter Four

Anti-Semitism and Anti-Discrimination in Private Law

Marc-Philippe Weller, Greta Göbel and
Markus Lieberknecht*

Introduction: Increasing Anti-Semitism in Germany

The number of reported cases of Anti-Semitism in Germany is on the rise. According to the RIAS Reporting Office[1] annual report and the Federal Ministry of the Interior's statistics on politically motivated crime[2], there are currently more anti-Semitic incidents than at any

*Prof. Dr. Marc-Philippe Weller, Licencié en droit (Montpellier), is Director at the Institute of Comparative Law, Conflict of Laws and International Business Law at Heidelberg University. Greta Göbel is an Academic Assistant and Senior Researcher at this Institute and is involved in the BMBF research project "Anti-Semitism as a Challenge for the Judiciary" (AS Just), which is being conducted in cooperation with the Universities of Gießen, Berlin (Humboldt), Potsdam and with the RIAS as well as with the Heidelberg High Court. Prof. Dr. Markus Lieberknecht, LL.M. (Harvard) used to be a Post-doc at Heidelberg University and is now Assistant Professor at the University of Osnabrück.

The article goes back to a lecture by Marc-Philippe Weller in the context of the Otto Meyerhof Ring Lecture at Ruperto Carola in the summer semester of 2021, building on the essay Weller/Lieberknecht, "Antisemitismus – Antworten des Privatrechts" in Juristenzeitung (JZ) 2019, 317-326, parts of which are reproduced below in an updated form, and supplementing it with more recent developments in private law with regard to anti-Semitism and anti-discrimination.

[1] Annual Report 2020 of the Bundesverband RIAS e.V.: https://www.report-antisemitism.de/documents/Antisemitische_Vorfaelle_in_Deutschland_Jahresbericht_RIAS_Bund_2020.pdf (last accessed 07.09.2021). Annual Report 2020 of the Bundesverband RIAS e.V.: https://www.report- antisemitism.de/documents/Antisemitische_Vorfaelle_in_Deutschland_Jahresbericht_RIAS_Bund_2020.pdf (last accessed 07.09.2021).

[2] Politically Motivated Crime in 2020, Nationwide Case Numbers, Federal Criminal Police Office, https://www.bmi.bund.de/SharedDocs/ downloads/ DE/veroeffentlichungen/2021/05/pmk-2020-bundesweite-fallzahlen.pdf?blob=publicationFile&v=4 (last accessed 07.09.2021).

time in the last 20 years.[3] Spikes in the statistics are mostly explained by a renewed intensification of the Middle East conflict between Israel and Palestine.[4] In addition, a constant increase has been noted since 2020 - the COVID-19 pandemic and conspiracy theories related to it are cited as the reason.[5]

Legislators reacted to this development primarily in the area of criminal law: in view of the increase in anti-Semitic crimes, the Law to Combat Right-Wing Extremism and Hate Crime[6] was passed. Among other things, this is intended to amend the rules on sentencing under Section 46 of the Criminal Code so that anti-Semitic motives on the part of perpetrators are to be considered in order to increase the severity of punishment. This is the first time that the term "anti-Semitic" has been used in a German law.[7]

---

[3] An accusatory overview of the current situation of Jews in Germany is given by Steinke, Terror gegen Juden, Wie antisemitische Gewalt erstarkt und der Staat versagt. Eine Anklage, Berlin 2020.

[4] This can also be seen in Baden-Württemberg in connection with the escalations in May 2021; there were increased attacks on synagogues and Jewish cemeteries, e.g., in Mannheim and Ulm: https://www.swr.de/ swraktuell/baden-wuerttemberg/ sorge-wegen-angriffe-auf-synagogen- auch-in-baden-wuerttemberg-100.html (last accessed 07.09.2021).

[5] Thus Botsch, Wetzel, Rasumny, https://mediendienst-integration.de/ artikel/ immer-mehr-antisemitische-straftaten.html (last accessed 07.09.2021) and also the 2020 annual report of the RIAS e.V. federal association: https://www.report-antisemitism. de/documents/Antisemitische_Vorfaelle_in_Deutschland_Jahresbericht_RIAS_ Bund_2020.pdf, p. 4 (last accessed 07.09.2021). Conspiracy theories and anti-Semitism are often closely linked, for example, many conspiracy myths contain anti-Semitic content (for example, the existence of a "directing power," which is then often equated with Judaism), Schnurr, Worüber sprechen wir eigentlich hier?, SPIEGEL Geschichte No. 3/2021, 28; according to Salzborn: "Anti- Semitism, as a cognitive and emotional system, aims at an ideological claim to all-explanation: as a worldview, it offers an all-encompassing system of resentments and (conspiracy) myths that were and are changeable in their concrete formulation. They are always directed against Jews, since anti-Semitism is based on projections and, as Theodor W. Adorno (1951: 125) put it, "rumors about the Jews."", https://www.bpb.de/politik/ extremismus/ antisemitismus/307644/was-ist-moderner-antisemitismus (last accessed 07.09.2021).

[6] Draft law of 30.03.2021, BGBl. I 2021, No. 13.

[7] The amendment was made in response to the attack on the synagogue in Halle, according to Liebscher, Pietrzyk, Lagodinsky, Steinitz, NJOZ 2020, 897, 897.

But what is legally meant by this term? And how can the law, especially civil law, which has been largely overlooked in this regard, counter it and contribute to combating anti-Semitism? These questions will be explored in the following.

"Anti-Semitism" in Private Law?

1. Attempt to Clarify the Term "Anti-Semitism"

Anti-Semitism is not easy to define in legal terms.[8] In the words of Israeli historian Moshe Zimmermann, the term is "so common that the question of its origin does not even seem to arise"[9].

The lack of clarity begins with the term itself, since it is a neologism that terminologically should refer to members of the Semitic language area - and thus also to Ethiopians and Arabs.[10] In fact, however, since its emergence in the late 19th century, it has denoted a negative

---

[8] Distinction between the levels of attitudes and those of actions also in Unabhängiger Expertenkreis Antisemitismus, BT-Drs. 18/11970, p. 24 ff; distinction of manifestations in individuals, culture and actions in Fein, Dimensions of Antisemitism: Attitudes, Collective Accusations and Actions, in: Fein (ed.), The Persisting Question: Sociological Perspectives and Social Contexts of Modern Anti-Semitism, Vol. 1, 1987, p. 67; inner attitudes are of particular relevance in private law, e.g., discrimination under the AGG, immorality, and violations of personality rights. This circumstance can lead to particular evidentiary difficulties, which is why, for example, the AGG contains a special easing of the burden of proof in § 22 AGG. For an application of the rule to all civil law claims based on unlawful discrimination, Thüsing, in: MüKo BGB, 9th ed. 2021, § 22 AGG Rn. 5.

[9] Moshe Zimmermann, in: Büttner (ed.), FS Werner Jochmann, vol. 1, 1986, 59.

[10] The Semitic language family includes Hebrew, Phoenician, Aramaic, Arabic, and various Ethiopian and South Arabic languages, Goldenberg, Semitic Languages, 2013, 10 ff.

attitude toward Jewish people alone.[11] Based on the usage of the term and in order to characterize the present-day manifestations of interest here, it is advisable to follow the broad understanding of the term,[12] which is unanimously shared in the literature, and to differentiate between internal conditions and external manifestations.[13]

The internal condition of anti-Semitism can be defined as a hostile attitude toward Jewish people as a collective. Rooting this attitude

---

[11] Berger Waldenegg, Was meint und wie erkennt man "Antisemitismus"? - Eine Begriffserklärung, in: Ansorge (ed.), Anti-Semitism in Europe and the Arab World, 2006, pp. 31, 34 f.

[12] Cf. the working definition of the International Holocaust Remembrance Alliance (IHRA), an international organization of which Germany has been a member state since its founding in 1998: "[...] a certain perception of Jews, which can be expressed as hatred towards Jews. Anti-Semitism is directed in word and deed against Jewish or non-Jewish individuals and/or their property, as well as against Jewish communal institutions and religious bodies. In addition, the State of Israel, understood in this context as a Jewish collective, can also be the target of such attacks," available at https://www. holocaustremembrance.com/de/node/196 (last accessed 07.09.2021); the IHRA working definition was used, for example, by LG München I in Urt. v. 19.1.2018, Az. 25 O 1612/17, Melzer/Knobloch, juris para. 77 and Urt. v. 10.12.2014, Case No. 25 O 14197/14, juris para. 71, Elsässer/ Ditfurth; see also Report of the Independent Group of Experts on Anti-Semitism, BT-Drs. 18/11970, p. 24: "Collective term for all attitudes and behaviors that impute negative characteristics to individuals, groups or institutions perceived as Jews on the basis of this affiliation."; see also Benz, Was ist Antisemitismus? 2004, p. 235: "[...] the totality of anti-Semitic statements, tendencies, resentments, attitudes, and actions regardless of their religious, racial, social, or other motives."; Fein, Dimensions of Antisemitism: Attitudes, Collective Accusations and Actions, in Fein (ed.), The Persisting Question: Sociological Perspectives and Social Contexts of Modern Antisemitism, Vol. 1, 1987, p. 67: "[...] a persisting latent structure of hostile beliefs toward Jews as a collectivity [...]"; Holz, Die Gegenwart des Antisemitismus, 2005, p. 10: "[...] a specific semantics in which a national, racial, and/or religious self-image is accompanied by a pejorative image of Jews."

[13] Distinction between the levels of attitudes and those of actions also in Unabhängiger Expertenkreis Antisemitismus, BT-Drs. 18/11970, p. 24 ff; distinction of manifestations in individuals, culture and actions in Fein, Dimensions of Antisemitism: Attitudes, Collective Accusations and Actions, in: Fein (ed.), The Persisting Question: Sociological Perspectives and Social Contexts of Modern Anti-Semitism, Vol. 1, 1987, p. 67; inner attitudes are of particular relevance in private law, e.g., discrimination under the AGG, immorality, and violations of personality rights. This circumstance can lead to particular evidentiary difficulties, which is why, for example, the AGG contains a special relief of the burden of proof in § 22 AGG. For an application of this rule to all civil law claims based on unlawful discrimination, cf. Thüsing, in: MüKo BGB, 9th ed. 2021, § 22 AGG Rn. 5.

in religious resentment is possible, but it can hardly be distinguished from hostility toward the group of Jews as a "race" and ethnic group.[14]

To be distinguished from anti-Semitism is criticism of the state of Israel (and its policies), which is often subsumed under the term anti- Zionism.[15] Admittedly, the literature emphasizes that anti-Zionism, in view of Israel's Jewish[16] and its national identity as the "home of the Jewish people"[17], at least often goes hand in hand

---

[14] Grünberger, Personale Gleichheit, 2013, p. 564; race and ethnic origin are particularly sensitive categories, they are "at the top of the civil law discrimination hierarchy", Grünberger, loc. cit. 706. A separation between the two characteristics is hardly possible and not very appropriate, cf. Baumgärtner, in: BeckOGK, status 1.6.2021, § 1 AGG Rn. 69 with further references from the case law of the ECJ and ECtHR. It is not possible to divide people into "races", on the historical development and meaning of the concept of "race", cf. Geulen, Der Rassenbegriff, in: Foroutan/Geulen/Illmer/Vogel/Wernsing (eds.), Das Phantom "Rasse", Bonn 2018. Also the concept of "ethnic origin" is partly seen as a continuation of an unjustified distinction and wrong focus on "affiliations", cf. Liebscher, Sind Juden weiß? Völkerrechtsblog Feb. 14, 2018, https://voelkerrechtsblog.org/de/sind-juden-weis/ (last accessed Sept. 13, 2021). On the idea and goal of postcategorical antidiscrimination law, cf. Liebscher, Rasse im Recht - Recht gegen Rassismus, Berlin 2021. Note also the discussion on whether the term "race" should be removed from the Basic Law, https://www.bundestag.de/dokumente/textarchiv/2020/ kw48-de-rassismus-807790 (last accessed 13.09.2021).

[15] Instructive Müller, Von Antizionismus und Antisemitismus - Stereotypbildung in der arabischen Öffentlichkeit, in: Ansorge (ed.), Antisemitismus in Europa und in der arabischen Welt, 2006, 163 ff.

[16] According to the official Israeli census, 74.5% of Israel's population in 2018 belonged to the Jewish religion, see Central Bureau of Statistics (CBS), Table 2.2 of 4.9.2018 (Population, by religion).

[17] The scope of the Jewish character of the state is controversially discussed in Israel. Testimony to this is provided, for example, by the quasi-constitutional Nation-State Law passed in 2018, which states, among other things, "The State of Israel is the nation-state of the Jewish people [...]. The exercise of the right to national self-determination in the State of Israel is unique to the Jewish people."; cf. in contrast the founding declaration of the State of Israel: "[The State of Israel] will promote the development of the land for the benefit of all its inhabitants; [...] it will secure to all its inhabitants, without distinction of religion, race or sex, complete equality of social and political rights; it will guarantee freedom of religion, conscience, language, education and culture; it will protect the holy places of all religions [...].", Provisional Government of Israel, Official Gazette No. 1, 14.5.1948.

with anti-Semitism of the kind described above.[18] The question of when justifiable criticism of the policies of the state of Israel turns into illegitimate anti-Semitism must be evaluated on a case-by-case basis.[19]

2. Forms of manifestation of anti-Semitism in private-law relationships

Anti-Semitism manifests itself in a range of behaviors. From the perspective of private law, the relevant constellations in Germany can be roughly divided into three categories based on the protected interests involved.[20]

a) Attacks on the dignity and personal honor of Jewish People

The first group includes attacks on the dignity and personal honor of Jewish people in the form of anti-Semitic statements in private and public spaces, including the Internet.[21] This group of cases

---

[18] Cf. on the Arab region Müller, Von Antizionismus und Antisemitismus - Stereotypenbildung in der arabischen Öffentlichkeit, in: Ansorge (ed.), Antisemitismus in Europa und in der arabischen Welt, 2006, 163: "On the other hand, anti-Israeli or anti-Zionist criticism and agitation repeatedly mix with anti-Semitic stereotypes. [...] Against this background, anti- Zionism and anti-Semitism are often no longer, or only with difficulty, can be distinguished."; on criticism of Israel in Germany as an outlet for anti- Semitic "bypass communication," Decker/ Kiess/Brähler, Antisemitische Ressentiments in Deutschland: Verbreitung und Ursachen, in: Decker/ Brähler (eds.), Flucht ins Autoritäre, 2018, 179, 181 ff.

[19] Zechlin, KJ 54 2021, 31-46, provides a closer look at the tension and a matrix-based guide for classifying statements between justified criticism of Israel's policies and anti-Semitism.

[20] A distinction is made between attitudes, manifest attitudes in the form of private or public statements and actions, including attacks on institutions and persons, in the report of the Independent Group of Experts on Anti- Semitism, BT Drs. 18/11970, p. 24 et seq.

[21] Ludyga describes in which cases a violation of the general right of personality is to be assumed, Ludyga, ZUM 2020, 440, 442 et seq.

ranges from anti-Semitic chants by soccer[22] spectators to derogatory, insulting statements against Jews[23]and the dissemination of fake news and conspiracy theories, including the denial or relativization of the Holocaust.[24]

b) Attacks on property, life or limb of Jewish people

The second group of cases consists of attacks on the property or even life and limb of Jewish people, i.e., anti-Semitically motivated hate crimes in the form of physical attacks[25] or vandalism[26].

---

[22] For example, German jurisprudence regularly deals - with inconsistent and sometimes remarkably lenient results - with the so-called "subway song" featuring a subway train either from Jerusalem or the city of the opposing team to Auschwitz, cf. OLG Hamm, decision dated Oct. 1, 2015, file no. III-1 RVs 66/15; OLG Rostock, decision dated July 23, 2007, file no. 1 Ss 080/06 I 42/06; LG Potsdam, Urt v. 21.2.2017, Az. 27 Ns 73/16; Cottbus, Beschl. v. 26.2.2009, Az. 24 Qs 411/08; on club liability for discriminatory behavior of soccer spectators cf. Weller/Benz/Wolf, JZ 2017, 237, 239; furthermore on anti-Semitism in German soccer cf. the report of the Independent Expert Group on Anti-Semitism, BT Drs. 18/11970, p. 272 ff.

[23] For more details, see infra VI. 3.

[24] The anchoring in untrue facts is so constitutive for anti-Semitism that Adorno characterizes it altogether as "the rumor about the Jews," Adorno, Minima Moralia, 1951, p. 200; on the historically most effective example of this, cf. Benz, Die Protokolle der Weisen von Zion, 2007, p. 108: "The 'Protocols' have long been the reference document of anti-Semitism par excellence. No other text has had a greater impact than the forged work on the Jewish world conspiracy [...]."; on the legal reappraisal of the "Protocols" in the so-called "Berne Trial," Bronner, Ein Gerücht über die Juden, 1999, pp. 135 ff. ; on Holocaust denial as a special form of dissemination of untrue facts (negationism) particularly worthy of punishment Matuschek, Erinnerungsstrafrecht, 2012, p. 36 ff.; cf. furthermore the ECHR's assessment that Holocaust denial is not protected by Art. 10 ECHR because invoking freedom of expression in this context constitutes an abuse of ECHR rights under Art. 17 ECHR, ECtHR, Judg. v. 20.10.2015, Case 25239/13, Dieudonné.

[25] The statistics show between 28 and 64 acts of violence with an anti-Semitic background for the years 2001-2015. Much debate was recently sparked by the belt attack on a kippa wearer in Berlin by a 19-year-old Syrian, whom the AG Tiergarten sentenced to four weeks of youth detention and a guided tour at the House of the Wannsee Conference, cf. Gehrke, Attacke auf Kippa-Träger: 19-Jähriger zu Arrest verurteilt, in Tagesspiegel, 25.6.2018, available at https://www.tagesspiegel.de/berlin/prozess-um-antisemitischen-angriff-in-berlin-attacke-auf-kippa-traeger-19-jaehriger- zu-arrest-verurteilt/22734120.html (last accessed 07.09.2021).

[26] Statistics were collected on 614 desecrations of Jewish cemeteries in 2001-2014 and 138 attacks on synagogues in 2008-2014 alone, Report of the Independent Panel of Experts on Anti-Semitism, BT Drs. 18/11970, p. 44 f. (Figs. III.6 and III.7).

c) Attacks on economic participation

Third, attacks on economic participation by attempting to oust[27] Jews from legal transactions, for example, by refusing to conclude legal transactions or subsequent withdrawal from contracts, especially in connection with calls for boycotts by private actors[28] and foreign boycott laws[29].

---

[27] The boycott of Jewish business activity inevitably evokes associations with the economic marginalization of the Jewish population in the early days of the Nazi era, instructive Barkai, Vom Boykott zur "Entjudung," 1988, p. 7: "The discriminatory measures against Jews living in Germany, which began immediately after the seizure of power on January 30, 1933, were aimed in particular at their economic activity. [...] As long as more drastic means were not yet enforceable, the National Socialist leadership saw the economic boycott, which was intended to undermine the material livelihood of the Jews, as the most effective means of persuading them to leave their homeland."

[28] A controversial example is the anti-Israeli so-called BDS campaign, for more details see infra VI. 3. c).

[29] For instance, the Kuwaiti boycott law dates back to a centrally orchestrated boycott campaign initiated by the Arab League since the 1940s, cf. Turck, Foreign Affairs 55 (1977) 472 et seq.; trade bans on its own citizens with Israelis apply (formally) in Qatar, Saudi Arabia, as well as Bangladesh; Lebanon maintains even more extensive boycott measures, cf. Weiss, Arab League Boycott of Israel, Congressional Research Service Report 7-5700 of Aug. 25, 2017, p. 2 et seq. The United Arab Emirates enacted Federal Decree Law No. 4 of 2020 on Aug. 29, 2020, repealing the former boycott law (Federal Law No. 15 of 1972 on the Boycott of the State of Israel) and entered into diplomatic negotiations with Israel, https://www.loc. gov/item/global-legal-monitor/2020-09-09/united-arab-emirates-new- decree-law-abolishes-law-on-boycott-of-israel/ (last accessed 13.09.2021). Bahrain, Sudan, and Morocco also entered into peace negotiations with Israel in 2020 and lifted boycott measures, https://www.bbc.com/ news/world-middle-east-54589235 (last accessed 13.09.2021), https:// www.aljazeera.com/news/2021/4/6/sudanese-cabinet-votes-to-repeal-israel-boycott-law (last accessed 13.09.2021), https://www. nytimes. com/2020/12/10/world/middleeast/israel-morocco-trump.html (last accessed 13.09.2021).

3 Example: Kuwait Airways

a) Decisions of the courts: LG Frankfurt, OLG Frankfurt, OLG Munich[30]

However, the difficulty private law has had so far in dealing with anti-Semitic phenomena becomes clear when looking at the "Kuwait Airways" case, which was brought before the Frankfurt Regional Court and the Munich Higher Regional Court. Neither the Regional Court[31] (LG) and the Higher Regional Courts[32] (OLG) nor the prevailing scholarly opinion[33] have been able to come up with a convincing answer to the Boycott Law No. 21/1964 of the State of Kuwait. This law prohibits Kuwaiti citizens from concluding contracts with Israelis. Citing this prohibition, Kuwait Airways refused to carry an Israeli citizen from Frankfurt to Bangkok (or from Frankfurt to Sri Lanka) with a stopover in Kuwait. The courts resort - without any convincing justification - to factual impossibility, saying that the law cannot get past facts: Kuwait does not allow the Israeli to enter or continue his journey anyway.[34]

---

[30] LG Frankfurt, Urt. v. 16.11.2017, Ref. 2-24 O 37/17 = JZ 2018, 153; OLG Frankfurt, Urt. v. 25.9.2018, Ref.: 16 U 209/17; OLG Munich, Judgment v. 24.6.2020, Az. 20 U 6415/19.

[31] LG Frankfurt, Urt. v. 16.11.2017, Az. 2-24 O 37/17 = JZ 2018, 153.

[32] OLG Frankfurt, Urt. v. 25.9.2018, Az.: 16 U 209/17; OLG München, Urt. v. 24.6.2020, Az. 20 U 6415/19.

[33] Mankowski, TranspR 2018, 104 ff.; Mörsdorf, JZ 2018, 156 ff.; Tonner, NJW 2018, 3595 f.

[34] OLG Frankfurt, Urt. v. 25.9.2018, Az.: 16 U 209/17, juris-Rn. 53 ff.; Mankowski, TranspR 2018, 104, 105 f.; OLG München, Urt. v. 24.6.2020, Az. 20 U 6415/19 = BeckRS 2020, 15428, Rn. 31 ff.

Is our private law really incapable of countering such anti-Semitic statutes - even if they originate in a foreign legal system? The courts' argumentation does not hold water in several respects: First, procedurally, Kuwait Airways' actual impossibility is not sufficiently demonstrated and proven.[35] Apart from that, the issue ultimately concerns the normative question of how a legal system evaluates the facts. Thirdly, *Windscheid's* concept of a claim, which is the basis of civil law, is misinterpreted, as it differentiates[36] between collectability, actionability and enforceability and, in the case of enforceability - which is also subject to party disposition - also distinguishes between domestic and foreign enforcement. It remains unclear why a domestic judgment for performance in kind would not have been enforceable at the place of departure, Germany, under § 888 of the Code of Civil Procedure.[37] Fourth, and most importantly, the prevailing opinion does not take sufficient account of the fact that the Kuwaiti Boycott Law pursues anti-Semitic purposes.

---

[35] See also Mankowski, TranspR 2018, 104, 106 f. on the LG Frankfurt.

[36] Weller, Die Vertragstreue, 2009, S. 226 ff., 374 ff.

[37] Contrary to Mörsdorf, JZ 2018, 156, 160, this is not a justifiable act that could be enforced by substitute performance (Section 887 ZPO). Rather, passengers are concerned precisely with flying with a particular airline, because not only compensation claims under the Air Passenger Rights Regulation (EC) No. 261/2004, but also any claims for damages in the event of damage depend on this and on the flight route, as the Germanwings case impressively demonstrates, Weller/Rentsch/Thomale, NJW 2015, 1909 et seq.

b) Comparative law perspective

Kuwait Airways' anti-Israeli business practices have also been the subject of litigation abroad:

For example, an Israeli who had been denied boarding on a direct flight from New York City to London successfully filed a complaint with the U.S. Department of Transportation alleging violation of U.S. anti-discrimination law[38]. Kuwait Airways subsequently discontinued the affected service.[39]

A discrimination complaint filed by an Israeli in Geneva for refusal to issue him a ticket from Geneva to Frankfurt failed.[40] In Great Britain, on the other hand, an Israeli citizen who had unsuccessfully tried to purchase a ticket from London to Bangkok via Kuwait invoked the

---

[38] Specifically, the DOT relied on 49 U.S. Code § 41319 ("An air carrier or foreign air carrier may not subject a person [...] in foreign air transportation to unreasonable discrimination.") and U.S. anti-boycott legislation. It affirmed a violation with regard to flights to countries under whose law Israelis may also disembark, see U.S. Department of Transportation letter of Sept. 30, 2015, p. 3 f., available at https://www.transportation.gov/sites/dot.gov/files/docs/Kuwait-Airways-Letter-Sept-30-2015.pdf (last accessed 07.09.2021): "This is not an adequate justification for denial of boarding because the sanctions that allegedly compelled [Kuwait Airways'] conduct are part of a discriminatory statutory scheme. [...] Moreover, Kuwait's refusal to sell airline tickets to Israeli citizens on a route between the United States and another location may also constitute a violation of U.S. anti-boycott laws and regulations [...]. Therefore, we find [Kuwait Airways'] actions inconsistent with and potentially in violation of U.S. anti- boycott laws to be unreasonable under U.S. policy. Finally, we do not find that Kuwait's interest in enforcing its laws is greater than the United States' interest in enforcing its laws in this case."

[39] Discontinued has been the service from New York, but not U.S. service to or via Kuwait, see Mouawad, Kuwait Airways Drops Flights to Avoid Israeli Passengers, New York Times, Jan. 15, 2016, available at https://www. nytimes. com/2016/01/16/business/kuwait-airways-drops-flights-to-avoid-israeli-passengers.html (last accessed 07.09.2021).

[40] Discriminatory rule now also in Switzerland - Kuwait Airways abandons Israelis, Blick, 22.4.2018, available at https://www.blick.ch/news/ schweiz/westschweiz/anti-israel-regel-jetzt-auch-in-der-schweiz-kuwait-airways-laesst-israelis-stehen-id8286168.html (last accessed 07.09.2021).

prohibition of discrimination under sec. 29 Equality Act 2010[41] and, according to her own statements, recovered a "substantial sum" from Kuwait Airways.[42]

4. Interim assessment: Anti-Semitism as a challenge for private law?

The Kuwait Airways case shows: Not only criminal law and public law are called upon to prevent anti-Semitism. On the contrary, a common denominator of the aforementioned manifestations of anti-Semitism is disregard in the legal and social relations of *private individuals*.[43] This is a cause for concern: Anti-Semitism is on the rise in these legal and social relations. This illustrates the increased importance of private law in combating anti-Semitism.

Behavioral Control through Private Law

However, it is not self-evident that private law is activated to regulate social concerns. On the legal level, criminal law has been primarily used to sanction anti-Semitism in the German State.[44] In contrast to criminal law and public law, private law regulates the legal relationships between citizens.

---

[41] Section 29 Equality Act (Provision of services, etc.) reads in subsection 1: "A person (a 'service provider') engaged in the provision of a service to the public or a section of the public (whether for consideration or not) shall not discriminate against a person in need of the service by not providing the service to that person."

[42] The dispute was apparently settled, see UK Lawyers for Israel, Kuwait Airways pays damages to Israeli after refusing her a ticket, Aug. 7, 2018, available at http://www.uklfi.com/kuwait-airways-pays-damages-to-israeli-after-refusing-her-a-ticket (last accessed 07.09.2021).

[43] Structural anti-Semitism on the part of the state is fortunately not considered a significant problem in Germany today, according to surveys. By contrast, 84% of Jews living in Hungary, for example, consider anti- Semitism in political life there (which admittedly goes beyond state action) to be a "very big" or "fairly big problem," see European Union Agency for Fundamental Rights, Discrimination and Hate Crime against Jews in the EU Member States: Experiences and Perceptions Related to Anti-Semitism, 2014, p. 19 (Table 2).

[44] Thus, the new law against hate crime and the amendment to Section 46 of the Criminal Code also only concern criminal law.

In many areas of law, it has now been recognized that effective law enforcement is achieved by activating citizens as potential creditors. Just think of European law (*van Gend & Loos*[45]), antitrust law (*Courage*[46]and *Manfredi*[47]), international law (Human Rights Litigation[48]) and climate change law (Climate Change Litigation[49]). European law, for example, only grew into an independent legal system detached from international law when the European Court of Justice granted the millions of EU citizens, in addition to the Member States, the active legitimacy to enforce the fundamental freedoms.[50]Without *private enforcement*[51], these areas of law would be largely deprived of their practical effectiveness today.

We argue that private law, through its consistent activation, can make a significant contribution to the fight against anti-Semitism.

Valuations of the Overall Legal Order with Regard to Anti-Semitism - Contribution of Private Law to the Fight against Anti-Semitism

But how can private law be mobilized? Legislators have (so far) remained inactive in the area of private law with regard to regulations on anti-Semitism. However, courts must also consider the values of the overall legal system when applying and interpreting private law regulations.

---

[45] EuGH, Urt. v. 5.2.1963, Rs. C-26/62, Van Gend & Loos, ECLI:EU:C:1963:1.

[46] EuGH, Urt. v. 20.9.2001, Rs. C-453/99, Courage/Crehan, ECLI:EU:C:2001:465.

[47] EuGH, Urt. v. 13.7.2006, Rs. C-295/04, Manfredi, ECLI:EU:C:2006:461.

[48] Weller/Kaller/Schulz, AcP 216 (2016), 387 ff.; Wagner, RabelsZ 2016, 717 ff.

[49] Kahl/Weller (Hrsg.), Climate Change Litigation, München, Baden-Baden, Oxford 2021.

[50] EuGH, Urt. v. 5.2.1963, Rs. C-26/62, Van Gend & Loos, ECLI:EU:C:1963: „[...] according to the spirit, the scheme and the wording of the Treaty, Article 12 [is] to be interpreted as producing direct effects and conferring individual rights which the State courts are bound to respect."; on this judgment of the century Kohler/ Puffer-Mariette, ZEuP 2014, 696, 704 ff.

[51] On the dichotomy of private and public law enforcement comprehensively Kern, ZZPInt 12 (2007), 351 et seq.

It therefore remains to be asked what values the extra-private legal order contains with regard to anti-Semitism that must be considered in the private-law framework.

1. Equal treatment requirements in constitutional and international law

At the level of constitutional and international law, there is a phalanx of regulations aimed at protecting against discrimination:

The most authoritative evaluation at the level of German constitutional law is contained in Article 3 (3) sentence 1 of the Basic Law, according to which no one may be discriminated against or given preferential treatment because of his or her sex, descent, race[52], language, homeland and origin, faith, religious or political views. The indirect third-party effect of fundamental rights in private law is recognized today.[53] Since 2006, the AGG has complimented the constitutional protection against discrimination in civil law[54], initially in the case of so-called mass transactions[55] and, in accordance with Section 1 AGG, even beyond this in the case of discrimination on grounds of race and ethnic origin and religion, which is relevant here.[56] The equality

---

[52] A discussion has unfolded around amending the Basic Law and deleting the word "race"; Liebscher, Verfassungsblog 11.06.2020, https:// verfassungsblog.de/das-problem-heisst-rassismus/ (last accessed 07.09.2021), argues for the replacement.

[53] Fundamental from a private law perspective already Canaris, AcP 184 (1984), 201 et seq.; on the spectrum of opinion Heun, in: Dreier (ed.), GG, 3rd ed. 2013, Art. 3 Rn. 70 et seq.; Kischel, in: BeckOK GG, 47th ed. as of 15.05.2021, Art. 3 Rn. 93, 210; Langenfeld, in: Maunz/Dürig, GG, 94th EL January 2021, Art. 3 para. 1 Rn. 123 et seq.

[54] On the relativization of the question of indirect third-party effect through this Kischel, in: BeckOK GG, 47th ed. as of 15.05.2021, Art. 3 para. 210; Sachs, in: Isensee/Kirchhof (ed.), Handbuch des Staatsrechts, Vol. VIII, 3rd ed. 2010, § 183 para. 168.

[55] Pursuant to Sec. 19 (1) No. 1 AGG, the prohibition of discrimination under civil law covers the "establishment, performance and termination of contractual obligations under civil law which typically come into existence without regard to the person on comparable terms and conditions in a large number of cases (mass transactions) [...]" as well as insurance contracts, whereby, pursuant to (2) and (3), restrictions apply to the renting of residential premises as well as special relationships of proximity and trust.

[56] Pursuant to Section 19 (2) in conjunction with 2 para. 1 nos. 5-8 AGG, the prohibition of discrimination under civil law in these cases extends in particular

guarantees of Article 3 of the Basic Law are further reinforced by the protection of personality, honor and dignity from Article 2 in conjunction with Article 1 (1) of the Basic Law. Article 1 (1) of the Basic Law, insofar as it is not a matter of unequal treatment but of interference - especially by private individuals - with these rights.[57]

German constitutional law is supplemented by regulations under European and international law. A second (limited[58]) starting point for protection against anti-Semitism is thus the prohibition of discrimination (in particular) on grounds of race and national origin contained in Article 14 of the ECHR, which also binds the judiciary.[59]Even if no direct obligation of the Convention states to remedy discriminatory behavior by private parties[60]is inferred from Art. 14 ECHR, the prohibition of discrimination has an impact on German private law via the doctrine of Convention-friendly[61]interpretation.

---

to "goods and services available to the public, including housing" without the requirement of mass business, in more detail Thüsing, in: MüKo BGB, 9th ed. 2021, § 2 AGG no. 29. In-depth question of the extent to which the AGG also prohibits discrimination against Israeli citizens, Weller/Lieberknecht/Smela, ZfPW 2020, 419 ff.

[57] For an anchoring of the fundamental law (core) discrimination protection as a whole in the right of personal dignity Lehner, Zivilrechtlicher Diskriminierungsschutz und Grundrechte, 2013, p. 226 et seq.

[58] Art. 14 ECHR is an accessory provision, i.e., it prohibits discrimination only insofar as it affects the rights and freedoms otherwise recognized in the ECHR. By contrast, Article 1 Additional Protocol No. 12 to the ECHR has a non-accessory effect, protecting discrimination on the same grounds as Article 14 ECHR with regard to the enjoyment of any right laid down by law. Germany has signed the 12th Additional Protocol, but has not yet ratified it.

[59] Cf. only Grabenwarter/Pabel, EMRK, 7. Auflage 2021, § 17 Rn. 6.

[60] Thus Meyer-Ladewig/Lehner, in: Meyer-Ladewig/Nettesheim/von Raumer (eds.), ECHR, 4th ed. 2017, Art. 14 para. 4; for a subjective right conferred by Art. 14 ECHR Jarass, Charta der Grundrechte der EU, 4th ed. 2021. Aufl. 2021, Art. 21 Rn. 3; protection and guarantee obligations have so far only been recognized by the ECtHR in exceptional constellations, Lehner, Zivilrechtlicher Diskriminierungsschutz und Grundrechte, 2013, p. 253.

[61] Cf. BVerfG, decision of 14.10.2004, Ref. 2 BvR 1481/04 = NJW 2004, 3407.

Furthermore, the fundamental rights of the Union, in this case specifically the prohibition[62] of discrimination on the grounds of racial or ethnic origin in Article 21 (1) CFR, have an indirect third-party effect on the application of private law insofar as it involves the implementation of Union law.[63]

Finally, German law must be interpreted[64] in light of other treaty obligations to protect against discrimination, in particular the UN Convention on Racial Discrimination[65], the UN Civil Pact[66]and the UN Social Pact[67].

---

[62] Perner, Grundfreiheiten, Grundrechte-Charta und Privatrecht, 2013, p. 173 et seq.; Jarass, Charta der Grundrechte der EU, 4th ed. 2021, Art. 21 para. 4; at least for Art. 31(2) CFR, the ECJ has recently also affirmed direct applicability to private law relationships, ECJ, Judg. v. 6.11.2018, verb. Cases C-569/16 and C-570/16.

[63] Unlike Art. 14 (see footnote 62 above), the provision is not accessory, i.e., it protects the enjoyment of any rights, Jarass, Charta der Grundrechte der EU, 4th ed. 2021, Art. 21 para. 1; on the controversial question of whether state duties to protect can be derived from Art. 21 CFR, Rossi, in: Calliess/Ruffert (eds.), EUV/AEUV, 5th ed. 2016, Art. 21 para. 10.

[64] Of more historical than legal significance is the Luxembourg Agreement concluded on September 10, 1952 (Wiedergutmachungsabkommen between the Federal Republic of Germany and Israel and the Jewish Claims Conference), by which the Federal Republic of Germany for the first time committed itself to financial reparations for Nazi injustice and thus paved the way for the establishment of diplomatic relations with Israel; for more on this, see Wolffssohn/Brechenmacher, Israel, in: Schmidt/Hellmann/Wolff (eds.), Handbuch zur deutschen Außenpolitik, 1st ed. 2007, 506, 507 et seq.

[65] International Convention on the Elimination of All Forms of Racial Discrimination of 7.3.1969, Federal Law Gazette 1985 II 1234. The Convention opposes any discrimination based on race, color, descent, national origin or ethnicity.

[66] International Covenant on Civil and Political Rights of 19.12.1966, Federal Law Gazette 1973 II 1553. The UN Civil Covenant obliges the contracting states in Art. 20 para. 2 to legally prohibit advocacy of national, racial or religious hatred that incites discrimination, hostility or violence and contains in Art. 26 p. 2 a prohibition of racial discrimination.

[67] The International Covenant on Economic, Social and Cultural Rights of 16 December 1966, Federal Law Gazette 1973 II 1469, contains in Art. 2 Para. 2 a prohibition of racial discrimination that is almost identical in content to the UN Civil Covenant.

2. Protection of the Jewish religion through freedom rights

In addition to the regulations that aim to protect against discriminatory unequal treatment, there are also civil rights that protect against interference with the specifically religious aspects of Jewish identity[68]: namely Article 4 (1) and (2) of the Basic Law, Article 9 (1) and (2) of the European Convention on Human Rights and Fundamental Freedoms, and Article 10 (1) of the Charter of Fundamental Rights[69]. In this context, the areas of protection encompass both the *forum internum* and *externum* of the Jewish religion and personally both natural persons and communities of persons.[70]

The prominent position of Jewish communities has been underscored by the federal and state governments through state treaties, which have given them the status of public corporations and the privileges associated with them, such as the right to levy taxes.[71]

---

[68] The concept of "Jewish identity" is likewise highly controversial and has changed over time (for a brief overview and thoughts on "Jewish identity" over time, see Simon, Zum Problem der jüdischen Identität, in: Horch/ Wardi, Jüdische Selbstwahrnehmung - La prise de conscience de l'identité juive, Tübingen 1997). For the purposes here, however, no clarification of terms is to be attempted, but rather the particular attitude of the German legal system toward certain aspects of Jewish life, Jewish religion, and the history of Jews in Germany is meant.

[69] All of the above-mentioned prohibitions of discrimination, i.e., Article 3 sentence 1 GG, Section 19 AGG, Article 14 ECHR and Article 21 (1) GRCh, also protect against unequal treatment on the basis of the characteristic of religion.

[70] On Art. 4 GG Germann, in: BeckOK GG, 47th ed. as of 15.05.2021, Art. 4 Rn. 11 et seq, 29 et seq.; on Art. 14 ECHR Grabenwarter/Pabel, ECHR, 7th ed. 2021, § 22 paras. 109, 113 et seq.; on Art. 10 CFR Waldhoff, in: Calliess/ Ruffert (ed.), EUV/ AEUV, 5th ed. 2016, Art. 10 CFR paras. 7, 11; on the relevance for the application of private law exemplarily Jayme, Religiöses Recht vor staatlichen Gerichten, 1999, p. 28 et seq.

[71] On the historical development Robbert, NVwZ 2009, 1211 et seq.; the advantages associated with the status of a corporation under public law include "[...] inclusion in the system of state promotion of religion, in particular the right to levy taxes (Art. 137 VI WRV) and the ability to legislate and serve [...]. In addition, there is a variety of special rights, such as tax benefits and exemptions in the law on costs and fees, the requirement of consideration for religious community interests in construction planning and regional planning law, etc.", Quaas, NVwZ 2009, 1400, 1402.

3. The criminal law framework

Criminal law sanctions racially motivated acts, including those with an anti-Semitic background, to a special degree. For example, the offense of incitement to hatred under Section 130 (1) of the Criminal Code protects both public peace and the dignity of individuals[72] from anti-Semitic incitement and specifically criminalizes the approval, denial or trivialization[73] of the Nazi genocide in Paragraph 3. Paragraph 4 prohibits the denial, trivialization or approval of acts committed under National Socialist tyranny if the dignity of the victims of National Socialist tyranny is thereby violated.[74]

Section 130 (1) Nos. 1 and 2 of the Criminal Code protects[75] Jews living in Germany as part of the domestic population.[76] With regard to incitement to hatred against Israelis, a gap in protection is sometimes stated, because these people - if they live abroad - are not part of the domestic population.[77] Correctly, however, the facts of the case are also fulfilled if a foreign-related statement also indirectly incites hatred against members of the group[78] addressed

---

[72] Kühl, in: Lackner/Kühl, StGB, 29. Aufl. 2018, § 130 Rn. 1.

[73] The so-called "simple Auschwitz lie", Rackow, in: BeckOK StGB, 50th ed. 1.5.2021, StGB § 130 Rn. 1.

[74] Rackow, in: BeckOK StGB, 50. Ed. 1.5.2021, StGB § 130 Rn. 38, 41.

[75] Settled case law, cf. only BGH, Urt. v. 21.4.1961, Az. 3 StR 55/60 = NJW 1961, 1364; BGH, Urt. v. 26.1.1983, Az. 3 StR 414/82 = NJW 1983, 1205; BGH, Urt. v. 15.12.2005, Az. 4 StR 283/05 0 NStZ-RR 2006, 305.

[76] On the limitation to domestic protected goods by the historical legislator BT Drs. 12/6853, S. 24.

[77] Therefore, Beck/Tometten, ZRP 2017, 244, tend to favor an amendment of the law.

[78] Schäfer/Anstötz, in: MüKo StGB, 4. Aufl. 2021, § 130 Rn. 31.

who live in Germany. This will regularly be the case with anti-Semitic incitement against Israelis. Furthermore, Section 185 of the Criminal Code provides an instrument for punishing individual and collective disparagement with an anti-Semitic background.[79]

Recently, the Act to Combat Right-Wing Extremism and Hate Crimes of March 30, 2021[80], has amended Section 46 of the Criminal Code so that an anti-Semitic motive leads to an increase in punishment. Although anti-Semitism as a motive for a crime was already covered by the previous statutory standard as well, after the attack on the synagogue in Halle, the explicit mention of anti-Semitism should have a symbolic effect and lead to practical relief.[81] Whether an act is anti-Semitically motivated becomes relevant, on the one hand,

---

[79] On the weighing in the case of the mere designation as a Jew, BVerfG, decision of September 6, 2000, file no. 1 BvR 1056/95 = NStZ 2001, 26; on the disparaging, inaccurate designation as a Jew, BGH, decision of Nov. 29, 1955, file no. 5 StR 322/55 = BGHSt 8, 325. 29.11.1955, file no. 5 StR 322/55 = BGHSt 8, 325; on the designation as "Gypsy Jew" BVerfG, decision of 12.7.2005, file no. 1 BvR 2097/02; on the collective insultability of the Jewish population BGH, decision of 28.2.1958, file no. 1 StR 387/57 = NJW 1958, 599; BGH, decision of. 18.9.1979, file no. VI ZR 140/78 = NJW 1980, 45; on the realization of § 189 StGB (denigration of the memory of the deceased) by Holocaust denial BayObLG, Urt. v. 17.12.1996, Az. 2St RR 178/96; to the insult (in any case with sufficient information and contextualization no insult) by the relief of a "Jew sow" at a church, OLG Naumburg, Urt. v. 4.2.2020 - 9 U 54/19.

[80] BGBl. I 2021 S. 441.

[81] Liebscher, Pietrzyk, Lagodinsky, Steinitz, NJOZ 2020, 897 (897).

in criminal proceedings, because then the public interest regularly stands in the way of discontinuing the proceedings if it is a matter[82] of private prosecution[83] or so-called minor offenses[84].

Anti-Semitically motivated acts are therefore not petty offenses, but must be consistently prosecuted and punished particularly severely. If handled consistently[85], criminal law thus enables powerful punishment of anti-Semitic behavior.

---

[82] The assumption of an anti-Semitic motive leads to other consequences in other areas as well, e.g., in criminal justice or administrative law. See Liebscher, Pietrzyk, Lagodinsky, Steinitz, NJOZ 2020, 897 (897 f.).

[83] In the case of private prosecution offenses, according to Section 376 of the Code of Criminal Procedure, charges are only brought if this is in the public interest, which includes, for example, insult, simple bodily injury, coercion and damage to property, Section 374 para. 1 of the Code of Criminal Procedure; in this context, Section 86 para. 2 RiStBV: "As a rule, a public interest will exist if the legal peace is disturbed beyond the circle of life of the injured person and the prosecution is a current concern of the general public, e.g., because of [...] the racist, xenophobic or other inhuman motives of the perpetrator [...]."

[84] Pursuant to Section 153 of the Code of Criminal Procedure, prosecution may be dispensed with in the case of misdemeanors if the culpability of the offender would be considered minor and there is no public interest in prosecution. This is determined according to the same standards as for § 376 StPO, cf. Valerius, in: BeckOK StPO, 40th ed. as of 01.07.2021, § 376 Rn. 3.

[85] Critical of German prosecution and sentencing practice, however, Beck/ Tometten, ZRP 2017, 244, 245 f.; on the legal history, cf. Jahr, Antisemitismus vor Gericht, 2011, pp. 320 ff.

4. The Basic Law as a counter-draft to the National Socialist Dictatorship: Wunsiedel Decision of the Constitutional Court (BVerfG)

The Basic Law is a counter-draft[86] to the National Socialist dictatorship. The Wunsiedel decision[87], in which the BVerfG has already stated this in the guiding principles, shows that the emergence of the Basic Law from a historical responsibility leads to a special attitude towards anti-Semitism.

The protection of "Jewish identity" or the fight against anti-Semitism can be regarded as a fundamental value of the constitution. The concept of a fundamental value goes back to *Isensee*: it is an unwritten value that underlies the constitution and thus has constitutional status itself.[88]

The significance of this fundamental value can be seen in the Wunsiedel decision: as the burial place of Rudolf Hess, Wunsiedel was a regular venue for memorial marches by neo-Nazis and right-wing extremists. When these were banned by the municipality, those affected appealed to the BVerfG with a constitutional complaint against the ban on assemblies and against Section 130 (4) of the German Criminal Code (StGB), invoking the right to freedom of expression under Article 5 of the Basic Law - a fundamental right of particular importance for democracy. What could be held against them? In principle, special laws,

---

[86] Explicitly described by the BVerfG as follows: "In view of the injustice and horror that elude general categories, which the National Socialist rule brought over Europe and large parts of the world, and the emergence of the Federal Republic of Germany understood as a counter-draft to this, an exception to the prohibition of special law for opinion-related laws is immanent in Article 5 I and II of the Basic Law for provisions that set limits to the propagandistic approval of the National Socialist regime in the years between 1933 and 1945. [...] The Basic Law can be interpreted to a large extent as a counter-draft to the totalitarianism of the National Socialist regime, and its structure, down to many details, is designed to learn from historical experience and to rule out a repetition of such injustice once and for all.", BVerfG, decision of 4. 11. 2009 - 1 BvR 2150/08, Rn. 64, 65 = NJW 2010, 47 (51 f.).

[87] BVerfG, decision of 4. 11. 2009 - 1 BvR 2150/08 = NJW 2010, 47.

[88] Isensee, Ethische Grundwerte im freiheitlichen Staat, in: Paus (ed.), Werte – Rechte - Normen, 1979, 131, 134.

i.e., not general laws but laws that are directed against an opinion as such, are prohibited and thus not suitable to justify an encroachment on freedom of opinion[89]. However, something different applies with regard to anti-Semitism: the BVerfG ruled that German history forms a fundamental value that shapes identity and opposes anti-Semitism and right-wing extremism, thereby justifying an interference with freedom of opinion:

*"With regard to the National Socialist regime in the years between 1933 and 1945, however, Article 5 (1) and (2) of the Basic Law also permits interference by means of regulations that do not meet the requirements of a general law. In view of the **unique injustice** and horror which this rule under **German responsibility** brought upon Europe and large parts of the world, and the significance of this past **for the identity of the Federal Republic of Germany**, statements which approve of this can have effects **which cannot be considered solely in generalizable categories**. [...]*

*An **exception** to the requirement of generality of laws restricting opinions pursuant to Article 5 II of the Basic Law is to be recognized for provisions aimed at preventing propagandistic affirmation of the National Socialist rule of violence and arbitrariness between the years 1933 and 1945. The inhuman regime of this period, which brought suffering, death and oppression on an immeasurable scale over Europe and the world, has a counter-image **identity-shaping significance** for the constitutional order of the Federal Republic of Germany that is **unique** and cannot be captured solely on the basis of general statutory provisions."[90]*

---

[89] Schemmer, in: BeckOK GG, 47. Ed. 15.5.2021, Art. 5 Rn. 98 f.; For more details on the definition of general laws, especially with regard to the Wunsiedel decision: Grabenwarter, in: Maunz/Dürig, 94th EL January 2021, Art. 5 para. 1, para. 2 Rn. 121 ff.

[90] BVerfG, Decision of 4. 11. 2009 - 1 BvR 2150/08 para. 52, 64 = NJW 2010, 47 (49, 51), emphasis by the authors.

5. Other state action / political stance of the German State

In our opinion, a central role in the interpretation of private law is played by the German vouching for the right of the State of Israel[91] to exist, which has grown out of historical responsibility, and a lasting fundamental solidarity of the German State with the concerns of Jewish people. In the stock of German legal sources, one searches almost in vain[92] for a concise codification of these political maxims. However, it would seem artificial and abbreviated to (ostensibly) exclude them from the application of the law.

Rather, since the end of the Second World War, the government's efforts to protect Jewish identity have been constantly pursued across all temporal and party-political developments.[93] One can speak here of a petrified guideline[94] of German politics.

Its significance is exemplified by the ad hoc reaction of the legislature to a judgment of the Regional Court of Cologne, which had punished

---

[91] Cf. in the context of the Kuwait case outlined supra Mankowski, TranspR 2018, 104, 105: "Of course, one has in mind the famous words of Chancellor Angela Merkel before the Knesset that Israel's security is part of the German reason of state. But has this fundamental foreign policy statement by the head of the executive branch also become the basis of German legislation? If one examines the German laws in this regard, one has to note an astonishing result: [...] Politicians have not followed their words with legal deeds. In the absence of a specific prohibition, the German courts are therefore thrown back on the use of general, non-specific instruments."

[92] The prohibition of boycott declarations in Section 7 AWV corresponds most closely to a measure law in support of Israel. There, however, a reference to the Arab League's boycott of Israel contained in the original draft law was deleted in favor of an open wording and (arguably) scope of application, cf. Pfeil/Mertgen, Compliance im Außenwirtschaftsrecht, 2016, ch. E. para. 154 et seq.

[93] For a comprehensive discussion of German-Israeli relations, see Wolffssohn/ Brechenmacher, Israel, in Schmidt/Hellmann/Wolff (eds.), Handbuch zur deutschen Außenpolitik, 1st ed. 2007, 506 ff.

[94] The frequently cited term "Staatsräson" (reason of state) is somewhat fuzzy because it refers to a state wisdom based on interests rather than values; for more on the history of ideas, see Crueger, Die außenpolitische Staatsräson der Bundesrepublik Deutschland, 2012, pp. 41 ff.

the religious circumcision of boys under criminal law.[95] Only a few months later, the legislature amended the German Civil Code (BGB) and, with § 1631d BGB, created a legally secure framework for performing *brit mila*.[96] The special respect for the Jewish rite is expressed in Section 1631d (2) of the German Civil Code, which also permits circumcision by medically qualified religious dignitaries.[97]

According to the thesis of this article, this basic attitude formulates a fundamental value not only of politics, but also of the *German legal system*[98]. This basic value becomes legally relevant as the result of a process that is described as a culture of remembrance[99]. This culture

---

[95] Cf. LG Köln, Urt. v. 7.5.2012, Ref. 151 Ns 169/11 = NJW 2012, 2128; the parents in the case in question were Muslims, but the legal opinion of the Cologne Regional Court had a de facto prohibitive effect in particular for the performance of the Jewish rite. Unlike its Muslim counterpart, the brit mila must be performed shortly after birth, i.e., when the child is not yet capable of giving consent, cf. Weller, Jewish Cultural Identity before German Courts, in: G. Stroumsa (ed.), Comparative Studies in the Humanities, Jerusalem 2018, pp. 223, 234.

[96] Weller, Jewish Cultural Identity before German Courts, in: G. Stroumsa (Hrsg.), Comparative Studies in the Humanities, Jerusalem 2018, S. 223, 231, 235 f.; the explanatory memorandum to the law deals in detail with the religious, historical and comparative legal backgrounds, cf. BT-Drs. 17/11295, S. 6 ff.

[97] Weller, Jewish Cultural Identity before German Courts, in: G. Stroumsa (Hrsg.), Comparative Studies in the Humanities, Jerusalem 2018, S. 223, 234 ff.

[98] On basic values as a legal category Isensee, Ethische Grundwerte im freiheitlichen Staat, in: Paus (ed.), Werte - Rechte - Normen, 1979, pp. 131, 134: "Pluralistic society requires a basic consensus above which the space of legitimate dissent opens up. The object of the necessary ethical consensus is the 'basic values'. The basic values embody that ethos in which the pluralistic society finds its unity."; on the increasing focus on basic values in civil law dogmatics Stürner, JZ 2012, 10, 15.

[99] Instructive on the term and the "ethical culture of remembrance" relevant here Aleida Assmann, Das neue Unbehagen an der Erinnerungskultur - Eine Intervention, 1st ed. 2013, p. 30 ff; a "collective learning process" is described by Bergmann, Antisemitismus in öffentlichen Konflikten, 1997, 502 ff; on the remembrance of the Holocaust as a legal postulate in public law and criminal law Matuschek, Erinnerungsstrafrecht, 2012, p. 118 ff.

of remembrance forms a universally agreed central narrative[100]in the state-political self-image of the German State. As a socio-political fundamental value, it can also have *legal* significance in the context of the interpretation of concepts of private law that are *open to interpretation.*[101]

This basic socio-political value does not bind the courts in the application of the law to the same extent as a legislative act, which the courts are obliged to follow strictly under Articles 20 (3) and 97 (1) of the Basic Law.[102] However, following the datum theory[103] developed by

---

[100] The conceptual proximity to the concept of "narrative norms" coined by Erik Jayme in private international law is quite intentional, instructive on this Schulze, Datum-Theorie und narrative Norm - Zu einem Privatrecht für die multikulturelle Gesellschaft, in: Jayme (ed.), Kulturelle Identität und Internationales Privatrecht, 2003, 155, 166 ff; on the role of narrative norms, namely the Washington Principles of Nazi-Confiscated Art, in the reparation of Nazi injustice Jayme, in: Becker (ed.), FS Manfred Rehbinder, 2002, 539, 543 ff.

[101] On the possibility of taking socio-political values into account in the context of interpreting legal concepts, cf. on "good faith" (Treu und Glauben) Olzen/ Looschelders, in: Staudinger, 2015, § 242 para. 142: "In general, this is intended to give "socio-ethical values" an input into the law. A regulation must thus be compatible with the ethics of rights immanent in the prevailing economic and social order, with the interests of the general public, with law and justice"; on "immorality" (Sittenwidrigkeit) Spindler, in: BeckOGK, 1.5.2021, § 826 BGB para. 4: "It does not depend solely on the actually existing practice within a certain [...] traffic circle, but on a minimum standard of social morality to be determined normatively. [...] In particular, the basic constitutional values in private law, which have been increasingly emphasised by the BVerfG, flow into the interpretation of the indeterminate concept of immorality.".

[102] Cf. Wilke, in: Isensee/Kirchhof (eds.), Handbuch des Staatsrechts, Vol. V, 3rd ed. 2007, § 112 Rn. 49: "In [Article 97 (1) of the Basic Law], the law is understood to be not only the formal law, but the totality of all legal norms. "; Hillgruber, in: Maunz/ Dürig, GG, 94th EL 2021, Art. 97 para. 55: "Interpretation is the method and path by which the judge explores the content of a legal provision, considering its placement in the overall legal order."

[103] When subsuming under the applicable substantive law (lex causae) under the law of reference (conflict of laws), the datum theory makes it possible to take into account the legal system(s) displaced by the law of reference in each case as well as values and principles of international law, comprehensively on this Weller, RabelsZ 2017, 747, 775 et seq.; same author, Die Datumtheorie, in: Gebauer/ Mansel/Schulze (eds.), Liber Amicorum Erik Jayme, 2019, 55 et seq, Die Grenzen der Vertragstreue von Krisenstaaten - Zur Einrede des Staatsnotstands gegenüber privaten Anleihegläubigern, 2013, p. 46 ff; Schulze, Datum-Theorie und narrative Norm - Zu einem Privatrecht für die multikulturelle Gesellschaft, in: Jayme (ed.), Kulturelle Identität und Internationales Privatrecht, 2003, 155, 156 ff.

Albert A. Ehrenzweig[104], we would like to put forward for discussion the thesis that the protection of Jewish life and Jewish identity as part of the petrified federal German executive maxim as well as an expression of the German culture of remembrance is not only of political but of *legal* significance. The protection of Jewish identity is to be considered in the application of law by German courts as a moral datum of the Federal Republic of Germany (following the *"domestic moral data-approach"* of *Albert A. Ehrenzweig*[105]) *firstly* in the context of the interpretation of the conflict of laws (*ordre public* and mandatory international laws) and *secondly* in the interpretation of the applicable substantive law. This will be outlined below for both levels by way of example.

Conflict of Laws Level: Private International Law

In matters with a foreign connection, private international law determines the law applicable to the case. Limits to the applicability of foreign law are found in *ordre public*. Irrespective of the reference to a certain law, so-called mandatory international laws are also applicable.

---

[104] Ehrenzweig, Buff. L. Rev. 16 (1966) 55 ff; ders, Private International Law, Vol. I, 3rd ed. 1974, p. 75 ff; on this Jayme, in: GS Albert Ehrenzweig, 1976, 35 ff; on the history of the development of the theory Jayme, Internationales Privatrecht - Ideengeschichte von Mancini und Ehrenzweig zum Europäischen Kollisionsrecht, 2009, p. 189 ff.

[105] According to Ehrenzweig, Buffalo Law Review 16 (1966), 55, 56, moral data (custom, usage, propriety, and other equitable pleas) are to be determined according to standards of the lex fori: "(...) I have spoken of moral data in those cases in which the law of the forum is automatically applied, notwithstanding the presence of foreign elements which would otherwise, according to recognized rules of choice of law, require the application of a foreign rule. In such cases, domestic rules formulated in the interests of justice and equity are applied. I have given as examples rules for acts committed with 'unclean hands' or 'with fraudulent intent'; acts that entail a forfeiture of rights; (...) I would contrast this automatic recourse to the law of the State of the forum as moral datum with the seemingly automatic reference to foreign rules as local datum."

1. Ordre public in the case of anti-Semitic content of the applicable foreign law

The *ordre public* of the *lex fori* serves as a "protective shield" of conflict of laws[106]against the realization of anti-Semitic values of foreign law. The protection of Jewish life and the commitment to Israel's right to exist are fundamental values of the German legal system. They are enriched by the prohibitions of discrimination in the ECHR and the CFR.[107]

The *ordre public* reservation does not provide for an abstract review of the content of the foreign norm, but focuses solely on the result in the individual case.[108] This flexibility, however, sufficiently enables the defense against anti-Semitic discrimination by a foreign *lex causae* even if they emanate from ostensibly neutral norms.

2. Mandatory international laws and anti-Semitism

Mandatory international laws become relevant from two different angles. On the one hand, it is necessary to deny effect to foreign mandatory norms with anti-Semitic content; on the other hand, domestic mandatory law can give effect to the value concepts of German law, regardless of the applicable lex causae.

a) Foreign mandatory law with anti-Semitic content

Anti-Israeli boycott laws such as the above-mentioned Kuwaiti Law No. 21/1964 are mandatory rules within the meaning of Article 9 (1) of the Rome I Regulation, because they claim applicability from the perspective of the issuing state due to its overriding political interests, irrespective of the law invoked by reference. In *international*

---

[106] In contrast to the institute of the right to intervene, which essentially has the positive function of applying legal norms by way of exception, the public policy reservation has only a negative defensive function, for more details see Voltz, in: Staudinger, 2013, Art. 6 EGBGB Rn. 8 ff. with further references.

[107] Martiny, in: MüKo BGB, 8. Aufl. 2021, Art. 21 Rom I-VO Rn. 3.

[108] Lorenz, in: BeckOK BGB, 59. Ed. Stand 1.8.2021, Art. 6 EGBGB Rn. 10f. However, an abstract control of the foreign law takes place according to a preferable view in the case of gender equality, cf. Art. 10 Rome III Regulation as well as Weller/Thomale/Zimmermann, JZ 2017, 1080 (theory of "cupiated referral").

contract law, Article 9 (3) sentence 2 Rome I Regulation leaves it to the discretion of the domestic court whether a foreign mandatory provision is to be given effect. The prerequisite, however, is that the norm originates from the legal system at the place of performance. This still echoes the "power theory", which in the earlier private international law considered the enforcement power of the issuing state of the mandatory provision as a criterion for the consideration of mandatory law.[109]

Boycott laws that contradict German fundamental values are *to be denied* application. The Kuwaiti boycott law, for example, is obviously based on anti-Semitic resentment, since its wording is directed "against Zionist gangs in occupied Palestine"[110]. Thus, in addition to its anti-Israeli agenda, it also reveals an anti-Semitic thrust.[111] Both aspects are incompatible with German *ordre public*. In contrast to the fact that the issuing state has the power to enforce its law on its territory, where the treaty is (also) to be fulfilled, the German value decision thus prevails at the level of referral.

The method of consideration, which comes into play only at the second (substantive) level, must be distinguished from the method of referral, which at the first (conflict-of-law) level of the so-called two-level theory of private international law calls a legal norm (with its facts and legal consequence) for application. This method makes it possible, within the framework of open legal concepts and general clauses of the *lex causae*, to consider as facts the legal rules of the

---

[109] Freitag, in: Reithmann/Martiny (eds.), International Contract Law, 8th ed. 2015, para. 5.114; in more detail on the power theory Busse, ZVglRWiss 1996, 386, 397 ff; Kuckein, Die „Berücksichtigung" von Eingriffsnormen im deutschen und englischen internationalen Vertragsrecht, 2008, 106 ff, each with further references.

[110] Quotation according to OLG Frankfurt, Urt. v. 25.9.2018, Az. 16 U 209/17, juris-Rn. 49.

[111] Thus also correctly the OLG Frankfurt, Urt. v. 25.9.2018, Case No. 16 U 209/17, juris-Rn. 44 et seq.: "Even taking into account these requirements - the nature and purpose of the encroachment provision as well as its consequences of application - the Kuwaiti encroachment provision, which can in principle be taken into account under Union law, is not to be given any effect. For this is unacceptable in terms of content according to German understanding."

displaced (deselected) legal systems under conflict of laws.[112] Its existence may still have *factual* effects (e.g., in the form of obstacles to performance), which may be subsumed under factual elements of law - such as impossibility or disturbance of the basis of the transaction. One then speaks of a consideration as a "date" on the level of substantive law.[113]

If the conditions of a (conflict of laws) reference according to Art. 9 (3) Rome I Regulation do not exist, such a (factual) consideration on the level of substantive law can still be considered.[114] However, the values of the forum, which oppose a conflict-of-law application of the foreign mandatory rule via the ordre public (Art. 6 EGBGB), must also be observed at the level of substantive law.[115] It is therefore important to avoid giving effect to the discriminatory content of mandatory rules, which may not be applied, via the "detour" of taking them into account in substantive law.[116]

b) Domestic mandatory law as corrective

A foreign lex causae - which, for example, could have been effectively agreed upon[117] in the Kuwait Airways case pursuant to Art. 5 (2) Rome I Regulation - can be overridden in contract law via Art. 9 (2) Rome I Regulation by the application of domestic mandatory rules.

This applies in particular to the AGG, whose norms, following Mansel, are correctly to be qualified as international mandatory

---

[112] Weller, RabelsZ 2017, 747, 770 ff.

[113] Weller, RabelsZ 2017, 747, 770 ff.

[114] EuGH, Urt. v. 18.10.2016, Rs. C-135/15, *Nikiforidis*, Rn. 50-52. On the application of this doctrine to individual norms of the BGB Riehm, in: BeckOGK, Stand 1.12.2018, § 275 BGB Rn. 358 f.; Freitag, NJW 2018, 430, 433.

[115] Weller, Die Datumtheorie, in Gebauer/Mansel/Schulze (eds.), Liber Amicorum Erik Jayme, 2019, 55, 80 et seq.

[116] For concrete application to the original case infra under VI. 1. b).

[117] Mankowski, TranspR 2018, 104, 107.

law[118]. In the non-contractual area, in particular if the mere initiation of the contract remains due to the discrimination, the same follows from Art. 16 Rome II Regulation.

The prohibition of boycott declarations according to § 7 AWV also represents a mandatory norm[119], so that German companies cannot effectively commit themselves to compliance with boycott regulations against Israel in foreign trade, irrespective of the lex causae.

3. Forced sales of Jewish art dealers

A comparative legal look at France shows: Here, too, private law contributes in the fight against anti-Semitism. The *Ordonnance n. 45-770 du 21 Avril 1945*[120], which was issued immediately after the end of the war, regulates the acquisition of works of art that Jewish art dealers were forced to sell.[121]

For the acquisition of these works, the Ordonnance stipulates the bad faith of all intermediary purchasers, so that no legal ownership of the works of art can be acquired - with the consequence that the heirs of the art dealers of the time can reclaim the paintings from the current owners. The *Cour de Cassation* (the French supreme court) applies the Ordonnance as mandatory law. The peculiarity of the cases is therefore that the Ordonnance applies "without any consideration of time and space"[122].

---

[118] Mansel, in: Heldrich et al. (eds.), FS Claus-Wilhelm Canaris zum 70. Geburtstag, vol. I, 2007, 809, 827; see also Pfeiffer, in: Jobst Hubertus (ed.), FS Peter Schwerdtner, 2003, 775, 786 et seq. ; Kocher, in: Witzleb et al. (eds.), FS Dieter Martiny, 2014, 411, 414 et seq.; Lüttringhaus, Grenzüberschreitender Diskriminierungsschutz – Das Internationale Privatrecht der Antidiskriminierung, 2010, 220 et seq.

[119] Weller, ZIP 2008, 857 ff.; also Freitag, in: Reithmann/Martiny (eds.), International Contract Law, 8th ed. 2015, para. 5.138; Martiny, in: MüKo BGB, 8th ed. 2021, Art. 9 Rome I Regulation para. 65.

[120] Ordinance no. 5-770 of April 21, 1945 on the second application of the ordinance of November 12, 1943 on the nullity of acts of spoliation carried out by the enemy or under his control and enacting the restitution to the victims of these acts of those of their property which were the subject of acts of disposal, available at: https://www.legifrance.gouv.fr/jorf/id/JORFTEXT000000522711 (last seen 07.09.2021)

[121] For more information on the Ordonnance: Jayme, IPRax 2021, 305 ff.

[122] Jayme, IPRax 2021, 305, 306.

4. Blocking Statutes as an instrument of defense

Another conceivable instrument would be a so-called Blocking Statute[123], which expressly declares foreign laws with anti-Semitic or anti-Israeli regulatory content to be undesirable and their observance to be unlawful, as well as granting those affected a claim for compensation for damages suffered in the event of violations.

De lege lata, Section 7 of the Foreign Trade and Payments Ordinance already stipulates a ban on boycott declarations.[124] However, this is limited to foreign trade law. Furthermore, Regulation (EC) No. 2271/96 is an instrument at the EU level, including a compensation provision, which is designed specifically to deflect undesirable foreign standards with extraterritorial application and is intended, for example, to block the Iran embargo of the USA with respect to EU companies that maintain business relations with Iran.[125] This regulation could be extended *de lege ferenda* to include anti-Israel norms. Nonetheless, apart from its symbolic character as a "narrative norm" (*Jayme*), the creation of a new regulation seems unnecessary given the legal instruments otherwise available.[126]

---

[123] On this, Basedow, Blocking Statutes, in: Basedow et al. (eds.), Encyclopaedia of Private International Law, 2017, 209 et seq.

[124] On the history of origins, see supra in fn. 85; that Section 7 AWV also has an individual-protective effect within the meaning of Section 823 (2) of the German Civil Code for Israeli contracting parties seems entirely justifiable.

[125] For more details, see Lieberknecht, IPRax 2018, 573 et seq.

[126] Arguably in favour, however, Mankowski, TranspR 2018, 104, 109 f.

Israel itself passed a law in 2011 to defend itself against anti-Israel boycotts.[127] This law grants affected parties a tort claim for compensation for causal damages[128] against individuals who have publicly called for a boycott of Israel. In the first case of application, a magistrate court in Jerusalem sentenced two New Zealand-based activists who had used an open letter to demand the cancellation of a planned concert by the singer Lorde in Tel Aviv. Based on the Anti-Boycott Law, three Israelis who had purchased tickets to the concert recovered the equivalent of several thousand euros in non-material damages against the anti-Israel activists and announced that the judgment would be enforced in New Zealand.[129]

Sanctioning of Anti-Semitic Behavior on the Level of Substantive Law

At the substantive law level, the fundamental values outlined above can be realized in several ways. First, the unrestricted participation of Jewish people in legal transactions must be guaranteed, and second, private law can sanction anti-Semitic discrimination. In this way, it can contribute to behavioral control and help to push back anti-Semitic behavior.[130]

---

[127] Law Preventing Harm to the State of Israel by Means of Boycott, 5711- 2011; German courts could at most apply this (intervention) law in the case of Israeli place of performance, Art. 9 para. 3 Rome I Regulation.

[128] The basis of the claim reads: "Anyone who intentionally calls for a public boycott against the State of Israel, where according to the content and circumstances of the call there is a sufficient probability that this call will bring about a boycott, commits a tort and gives rise to the applicability of tort law (new version), provided he is aware of this possibility." (own translation); A claim for non-pecuniary punitive damages in the case of intentional boycott measures, which was originally also included, was declared unconstitutional by the Supreme Court of Israel for violating the right to freedom of expression, cf. Supreme Court, Urt. v. 15.4.2015, verb. Az. HCJ 5239/11, HCJ 5392/11, HCJ 5549/11 and HCJ 2072/12, Avneri v. Knesset.

[129] Roy, Israel fines New Zealand women $18,000 for urging Lorde concert boycott, The Guardian vom 12.10.2018, available at https://www.theguardian.com/music/2018/oct/12/israel-fines-new-zealand-teenagers-18000-for-urging-lorde-concert-boycott (last retrieved on 07.09.2021).

[130] This is not about an additional penal function of the compensation, but about a (desired) preventive side effect of the compensation, on this Wagner, AcP 206 (2006), 352, 360 ff., 471 ff.; on the general right of personality Rixecker, in: MüKo BGB, 9th ed. 2021, Appendix to § 12 para. 296 ff.

1. Contract law

A party to a contract may not be permitted to withdraw from the contract or torpedo its performance by reference to the other party's Jewish origin. In this respect, Kuwait Airways could have neither contested the contract with the Israeli passenger nor successfully raised an objection or defense against its own obligation to perform.

a) Contestation

A mistake about the Israeli origin of a contractual partner does not constitute grounds for cancellation of the contract pursuant to Section 119 (2) Var. 1 BGB[131]. Conversely, in consistent continuation of the "Thor Steinar" jurisprudence of the Federal Court of Justice[132], the anti- Semitic attitude of one party may constitute a material contractual characteristic which entitles the other party to rescind the contract because the other party can then no longer be expected to perform the contract (further).[133]

b) Performance in kind

The principle of performance in kind[134], which applies under the German Civil Code, cannot be undermined by anti-Semitically

---

[131] The criteria of ethnic origin and religious affiliation are generally irrelevant when initiating a contract, Singer, in: Staudinger, 2017, § 119 para. 89; Weller/Grethe, ZEuP 2015, 606: Discrimination prohibition due to sexual orientation in hotel accommodation contracts.

[132] On voidability due to fraudulent misrepresentation by omission BGH NJW 2010, 3362 - Thor Steinar I: "In public, this trademark is exclusively associated with the radical right-wing scene"; BGH NZM 2010, 788 - Thor Steinar II, para. 18. 18: "The Court of Appeal rightly assumed that the defendant had fraudulently deceived the plaintiff by not informing the plaintiff prior to the conclusion of the contract of its intention to sell almost exclusively goods of the trademark 'Thor Steinar' in the rented premises."

[133] Cf. also BGH, Urt. v. 9.3.2012, Ref. V ZR 115/11 = JZ 2012, 686, according to which the fact that a hotel guest turned out to be the NPD chairman was not sufficient as a "particularly weighty factual reason" for a house ban on the part of the hotel during the agreed accommodation period, whereby the question of contestability was left open because there was a time limit pursuant to section 121 (1) BGB.

[134] On the development from monetary condemnation to performance in kind in substantive law Olzen, in: Staudinger, 2020, § 241 Rn. 25 ff.

motivated objections. Domestic courts must ensure that a party cannot take refuge in impossibility, unreasonableness or compensation for damages merely to avoid having to perform to Jewish contractual partners. This is exemplified by the handling of the Kuwaiti boycott law in the context of Section 275 of the German Civil Code.

Contrary to the Frankfurt Regional Court, a *legal* impossibility must be denied in such cases. This would be a recourse to the *normative* content of the boycott law. Such a recourse is excluded, because the inapplicability of the law as a mandatory law according to Art. 9 (3) Rome I Regulation "penetrates" to the level of substantive law.[135]

But even the subsumption under the facts of *actual* impossibility is open to normative evaluations at the level of actionability[136]. For example, German law does not recognize financial impossibility even if the debtor actually has no money.[137] Thus, under German law, actual impediments to performance may well be shifted from the actionability level to the enforceability level (insolvency law).

Contrary to the Higher Regional Courts of Frankfurt and Munich, the protection of Jewish identity as a moral datum of the Federal Republic of Germany prohibits the assumption of an actual impossibility if the debtor believes that it is unreasonable to expect it to service Jews. The justified interest of the plaintiff in the Kuwait case consisted in not being excluded from payment in kind as an Israeli under German law. What mattered to him first and foremost was to be recognized as the holder of an actionable claim. Whether the plaintiff later wishes to enforce a judgment for performance is (solely) at his discretion;

---

[135] Cf. on the whole supra V. 2. a); so also OLG Frankfurt, Urt. v. 25.9.2018, Ref. 16 U 209/17, juris-Rn. 37 et seq.; differently still the lower court, LG Frankfurt, Urt. v. 16.11.2017, Ref. 2-24 O 37/17, juris-Rn. 38 et seq. = JZ 2018, 153, 154; as here already Freitag, NJW 2018, 430, 433 et seq. ; probably also Mankowski, TranspR 2018, 104, 107; Mörsdorf, JZ 2018, 156, 159; on the methodological relevance of the referral barriers for the import of foreign "data" Weller, Die Datumtheorie, in: Gebauer/Mansel/Schulze (eds.), Liber Amicorum Erik Jayme, 2019, 55, 80 et seq.

[136] On the distinction between the enforceability of a claim (merits of the action) and its later enforceability Weller, Die Vertragstreue, 2009, p. 374 ff; on enforcement in kind Nehlsen-von Stryk, AcP 193 (1993), 529 ff.

[137] Weller/Harms, WM 2012, 2305 ff.

the court may not paternalistically anticipate this question. Whether the plaintiff can enforce a judgment for performance in kind with the help of state enforcement bodies depends on the applicable (possibly foreign) enforcement statute. Even if a judgment for performance in kind cannot be enforced in Germany (see, for example, Section 888 (3) of the German Code of Civil Procedure), this does not mean *eo ipso* that enforcement would not be possible in other countries either. The Higher Regional Court of Frankfurt and the Higher Regional Court of Munich anticipated these questions, which only arise at the enforcement level, by affirming the actual impossibility, thereby giving effect to the anti-Semitism orchestrated by the state of Kuwait.

2. Compensation under the AGG

Anti-Semitic discrimination can result in claims for compensation. An independent claim for compensation due to violations of the prohibition of discrimination under civil law pursuant to Section 19 AGG arises from Section 21 (2) AGG which grants a claim for material and immaterial damages for discrimination.[138] The claim therefore grants financial regress for serious non-material injuries[139], which must normally be granted in the case of anti-Semitically motivated discrimination.[140]

a) Direct discrimination

Discrimination against Jews can first be subsumed under the discrimination criterion of religion, insofar as religion-specific aspects are affected.[141]

---

[138] The existence of a contracting claim under section 21(1) AGG is controversial, but now largely recognised, cf. on this Thüsing, in: MüKo 8th ed. 2018, section 21 AGG para. 17 et seq. with further references.

[139] Thüsing, in: MüKo BGB, 9th ed. 2021, § 21 AGG para. 55: "A serious violation is to be assumed if the disadvantaged person has been 'degraded' and has been unlawfully deprived of the chances of equal participation in economic life solely on the basis of his or her 'being'"; more on the violation of the general right of personality infra under VI. 3. a).

[140] In detail on the possible sanctioning of anti-Semitic discrimination, see Weller/ Lieberknecht/Smela, ZfPW 2020, 419-432.

[141] Weller/Lieberknecht/Smela, ZfPW 2020, 419 (423).

In addition, the criteria of ethnic origin and race[142] can be considered - the Supreme Court UK[143] and some German courts[144] have assumed discrimination on the basis of ethnic origin in relevant cases of discrimination against Jews.[145]

The OLG Munich denied a hidden direct discrimination in the sense of § 3 para. 1 AGG because of ethnic origin (or religion): Such is only the case if "a distinction is made according to an apparently objective, non-discriminatory criterion, which, however, is inseparably connected with a characteristic mentioned in § 1 AGG and thus categorically exclusively affects carriers of a discriminatory characteristic"[146].

b) Indirect discrimination

However, indirect discrimination within the meaning of Section 3 (2) of the General Equal Treatment Act is possible due to the link to nationality. Nationality itself is not one of the grounds for discrimination listed in §§ 1, 19 AGG. However, since over 74% of the Israeli population is Jewish, it seems reasonable to assume that the discrimination against Israeli citizens constitutes at least indirect discrimination against Jews (on the grounds of religion or ethnic origin). According to the Federal Labour Court (BAG), it is sufficient for indirect discrimination if a supposedly neutral criterion (such as nationality) *regularly* disadvantages a religious community or an ethnic group. In view of the population composition of Israel, the

---

[142] Both terms are problematic and controversial. It is not a matter of an "objective assignment to a 'race'", but rather of the subjective perception of the discriminating person about a certain group and the affiliation of this person to this group: with further references Weller/Lieberknecht/Smela, ZfPW 2020, 419, 423 ff.

[143] UK Supreme Court, Urt. v. 16.12.2009 – [2009] UKSC 15, R (on the application of E) (Respondent) v Governing Body of JFS and the Admissions Appeal Panel of JFS and others (Appellants), Rn. 28.

[144] OLG Frankfurt a.M., Urt. v. 25.9.2018 – 16 U 209/17 = NJW 2018, 3591 (3595).

[145] Also Weller/Lieberknecht/Smela, ZfPW 2020, 419, 424; Thüsing, in: MüKo, 9th ed. 2021, § 1 AGG para. 21. Horcher, in: BeckOK BGB, 59th ed., status: 01.08.2021, § 1 AGG, para. 15, argues against this.

[146] OLG München, Urt. v. 24.6.2020, Az. 20 U 6415/19 = BeckRS 2020, 15428, Rn. 48; with reference to BAG, NZA 2014, 372 Rn. 72; BAG, NZA 2011, 1370 Rn. 23.

nationality- related characteristic "Israeli" also focuses on members of the ethnic group of Jews or members of the Jewish religion, which incidentally corresponds to the purpose of the Kuwaiti law.[147] The fact that Arab Israelis are also covered by the boycott does not prevent the assumption of indirect discrimination.[148]

The Munich Higher Regional Court leaves it open whether such indirect discrimination exists, but in any case, sees a justifying reason in the form of actual impossibility.[149] However, it must be countered with the above that the fact of actual impossibility also contains value elements and the debtor cannot invoke this here due to the underlying anti-Semitic boycott law. Thus, there is also no justifiable reason that would justify indirect discrimination.

It is also discussed - *de lege ferenda* - to include the criterion of nationality in the catalog of grounds of discrimination, so that in a case like this there would be direct discrimination.[150]

3. Tort Claims

a) The general right of personality

A violation of the general right of personality may give rise to various claims on the part of the injured party: On the one hand, claims for compensation based on Section 823 (1) of the German Civil Code (BGB) in conjunction with Articles 1 and 2 of the German Basic Law (GG) must be considered.

---

[147] An objective justification according to § 3 para. 2 AGG is ruled out according to the above; likewise Mörsdorf, JZ 2018, 156, 158 et seq.

[148] Cf. however the concerns in Mankowski, TranspR 2018, 104, 180 f.

[149] OLG München, Urt. v. 24.6.2020, Az. 20 U 6415/19 = BeckRS 2020, 15428, Rn. 50 f.

[150] Weller/Lieberknecht/Smela, ZfPW 2020, 419, 430 et seq., are in favour of this; because of the AGG's origin in Union law and its location in Art. 19 TFEU (instead of Art. 18 TFEU), they are probably more skeptical: Thüsing, in: MüKo, 9th ed. 2021, § 1 AGG para. 16.

aa) Anti-Semitic offenses

In addition to the protection of property and health, the general right of personality protected[151] under Section 823 (1) (and preventively by analogy with Section 1004 (1) of the German Civil Code) is a starting point for claims in tort. Pursuant to Section 21 (3) AGG, tortious liability is neither displaced nor modified by the claims regulated in the AGG.[152] Specifically, the protection against disparagement and distorting portrayal[153] may enable the affected person to seek monetary compensation[154] for anti-Semitic slights. Admittedly, case law sets high standards for the existence of a violation of personality[155]. However, in the case of anti-Semitic hostility, a violation of personality rights can generally be assumed from a German perspective in view of the severity of the taboo violation, especially when personal (family) fates are involved.[156] In this respect, the VI Civil Senate of the Federal Court of Justice clarified as early as the 1970s that generally held anti-Semitic statements in the form of Holocaust denial can at the same time constitute insults to every individual of Jewish descent.[157]

---

[151] Constant case law, cf. only BGH, Urt. v. 1.12.1999, Ref. I ZR 49/97 = GRUR 2000, 709 et seq.

[152] Tortious claims gain independent relevance in particular because they are only subject to the regular limitation period, which is generous in comparison to the two-month period under section 21 (5) AGG.

[153] Detailed Hager, in: Staudinger, 2017, § 823 Rn. C 63 ff.

[154] On this constitutionally recognised further development of the law despite the lack of a provision in § 253 BGB Lange/Schiemann, Schadensersatz, 3rd ed. 2003, p. 449 ff.

[155] Schiemann, in: Staudinger, 2017, § 253 Rn. 58 ff.

[156] However, the Frankfurt Higher Regional Court (OLG) rejected a serious breach on the grounds that the actual impossibility constituted an objective reason for the non-transportation, OLG Frankfurt, Urt. v. 25.9.2018, Case No. 16 U 209/17, juris-Rn. 69 et seq.; in our opinion, the fact that the Kuwaiti state was the sole shareholder behind the defendant and that a compensation payment would thus have economically affected precisely the author of the discriminatory law should also have been considered.

[157] Cf. the guiding principle in BGH, Urt. v. 18.9.1979, Ref. VI ZR 140/78 = NJW 1980, 45: "People of Jewish descent are entitled to recognition of the persecution fate of the Jews under National Socialism on the basis of their right of personality in the Federal Republic [of Germany]. Anyone who denies the murder of Jews in the 'Third Reich'. insults every one of them. Persons born after 1945 are also affected by such statements [...]."

bb) Accusation of anti-Semitism

However, the general right of personality can at the same time represent the line of defense of those persons who find themselves exposed to accusations of anti-Semitism.

This tension is revealed by a legal dispute in which the publicist Abraham Melzer sought an injunction from Charlotte Knobloch, the president of the Jewish Community of Munich and Upper Bavaria, to refrain from making the statement that he was "downright notorious for his anti-Semitic statements.[158] Knobloch's statement referred to remarks in which Melzer had compared functionaries of the Israeli state with National Socialist functionaries and had described slogans such as "Hamas, Hamas, Jews to the gas" as a "perfectly understandable reaction" to Israeli policy.[159] Even in view of the fact that Abraham Melzer is also Jewish, the Munich I Regional Court considered his statements to be anti-Semitic, thus making it clear that the limit of permissible criticism of Israel had been exceeded.

The cases of Jutta Ditfurth - Jürgen Elsässer[160] and Amadeu Antonio Foundation - Xavier Naidoo[161] were decided differently: there, the courts ruled that Elsässer and Naidoo may not be called anti-Semites, which led to great public criticism.[162]

cc) Cease and desist from anti-Semitic concerts

Furthermore, in addition to claims for compensation due to infringement of the general right of personality, claims for injunctive relief can also arise from Section 1004 of the German Civil Code by

---

[158] LG München I, Urt. v. 19.1.2018, ref. 25 O 1612/17; in a similar constellation, the Higher Regional Court of Munich prohibited the author Jutta Ditfurth from calling the neo-right-wing publicist Jürgen Elsässer an "ardent anti- Semite", OLG Munich, decision of 28.9.2015, ref. 18 U 169/15, Elsässer/ Ditfurth.

[159] LG München I, Urt. v. 19.1.2018, Az. 25 O 1612/17, juris-Rn. 13 ff.

[160] LG München I Urt. v. 8.10.2014 –25 O 14197/14, BeckRS 2016, 10888; OLG München Urt. v. 28.9.2015 – 18 U 169/15 Pre, BeckRS 2015, 128693.

[161] OLG Nürnberg, Urt. v. 22.10.2019 – 3 U 1523/18, ZUM-RD 2020, 274.

[162] Liebscher, Pietrzyk, Lagodinsky, Steinitz, NJOZ 2020, 897, 901 f.; Ludyga, ZUM 2020, 440, 446.

analogy, for example against a concert organizer in the case of anti-Semitic song lyrics.[163]

b) Norms of the German Criminal Code (StGB) as protective laws within the meaning of Section 823 (2) of the German Civil Code (BGB).

Anti-Semitic statements and behavior are covered by a number of criminal offenses, which in turn mostly represent individual-protective norms[164]. This opens up the possibility of a claim for damages under Section 823 (2) in conjunction with the relevant criminal law norm. Since property, health and honor violations as well as business-related interference are already compensable via Section 823 (1) of the German Civil Code, the additional protection is likely to be limited to pure financial losses.

The prosecution of civil claims for criminal statements on Internet platforms was also made easier in 2017 with the NetzDG. Insofar as it is necessary to enforce such claims, the respective operator of the Internet service must hand over the master data of the alleged tortfeasor to the injured party by court order pursuant to Section 14 (3) TMG, as amended.[165] The assertion of flanking civil claims in the criminal adhesion proceedings (sections 403 et seq. of the Code of Criminal Procedure) enables an efficient bundling of *public* and *private enforcement*.

---

[163] LG Saarbrücken, order of 5.12.2019 - 5 T 438/19 = ZUM-RD 2020, 551 et seq.

[164] See supra IV. 3.

[165] § Section 14 subsection 3 TMG refers to Section 1 subsection 3 TMG, the catalogue of which includes Section 130 StGB (incitement to hatred), Section 185 StGB (insult) and Section 241 StGB (threat). However, the provision of information requires a court order, Section 14 (4) TMG.

c) Boycott calls as immoral damage?

Privately initiated boycott campaigns against Israeli merchants meet the criteria of Section 826 of the German Civil Code (BGB)[166] if they are motivated by anti-Semitism[167]. In accordance with § 840 BGB, all persons who have contributed - for example, in the form of disseminating a call for a boycott - are jointly and severally liable for any damage.

Calls to boycott Israeli products, the most prominent example of which is the worldwide campaign known as BDS ("Boycott, Divestment and Sanctions"), represent difficult borderline cases.[168] The fact that such calls for a blanket boycott of Israel demand resolute opposition does not make them *eo ipso* illegal or immoral in view of the right to freedom of expression of critics of Israel under Article 5 (1) of the Basic Law.[169] Because a general evaluation of the campaign is already difficult due to its decentralized worldwide organization, it ultimately depends on an evaluation of concrete activities, which, as far as can be seen, has not yet been carried out by German courts.[170]

---

[166] In individual cases, such calls may be directly business-related within the meaning of Section 823 (1) of the German Civil Code in conjunction with the right to established and exercised business operations, for more details on the relationship to Section 826 of the German Civil Code see Oechsler, in: Staudinger, 2018, Section 826 para. 406 f. A claim under Section 4 of the German Unfair Competition Act is theoretically conceivable, but requires activities among competitors, for more details on the relationship see Wagner, in: MüKo BGB, 8th ed. 2020, Section 823 para. 398.

[167] See also Wagner, in: MüKo BGB, 8. Aufl. 2020, § 823 Rn. 401.

[168] The case described above under V. 4. also involved BDS activists.

[169] Fundamental to the role of Art. 5 GG in private boycott calls BVerfG, Urt. v. 15.1.1958, Case No. 1 BvR 400/51, Lüth = BVerfGE 7, 198; BVerfG, Decision of 26.2.1969, Case No. 1 BvR 619/63, Blinkfüer = BVerfGE 25, 256.

[170] A claim for municipal admission by BDS activists asserted in Munich already failed due to admissibility, VG München, Beschl. v. 7.2.2018, Az. M 7 E 18.451; in the above-mentioned Melzer/Knobloch case, the plaintiff's BDS activities were submitted but not used to justify the decision, LG München I, Urt. v. 19.1.2018, Ref. 25 O 1612/17, juris-Rn. 48, 63.

Outlook / Conclusion

On the basis of the starting points outlined above, it can be seen that private law offers numerous means of taking effective action against anti-Semitism. The historical responsibility to combat anti-Semitism in the German State, which underlies the German legal system, also finds its way into legal relations between private parties and must thus be considered by courts there as well.

Chapter Five

After Halle: Some Thoughts on the Situation of the Jewish Community in Germany

Frederek Musall

> "That's enough, I've had it up to here/
> I've lost my vision, I've lost my hope"
> - Maximo Park, "Graffiti"

I.

I am writing these lines one day after Yom Kippur. Two years after the attack in Halle. And barely 24 hours after a foiled attack on the Jewish community in Hagen. Perhaps I should just take my hands off the keyboard and leave it at this brief statement, because basically everything that could be said seems to have been said. Namely, how little has actually changed in this country. After Halle.

In the very year in which 1700 years of Jewish life in Germany are celebrated in many places with great expense and the WDR program "Freitagnacht Jews" wins - quite rightly, by the way - the German Television Prize, the very life of Jews in Germany is endangered as rarely before in recent years. Public debates about whether the primary threat comes from right-wing extremists, Islamists or Israel-haters say a lot about identity politics, discourses and lines of conflict, but in practice they are of little help to those affected by anti-Semitic violence. Rather, the impression is that anti-Semitism is talked about in public, but hardly ever with those affected by it, let alone that they are really listened to. This would be important to prevent them from experiencing yet another moment of discrimination and marginalization, namely not being able to provide information about their experiences. For anti-Semitism in Germany is not something that can be measured on the basis of attacks alone. Anti-Semitism is something that Jews in this country encounter on a daily basis and in many different forms. In schoolyards, on the sports field, at work, on social media, on the Internet. From Islamists and anti-Zionists, from leftists and rightists, from Internet trolls. And not infrequently from the middle of society.

II.

Thus, the attack in Halle was by no means as surprising for many Jews as it was for the rest of the population, as Central Council President Dr. Josef Schuster, among others, made clear barely 24 hours later on the occasion of the ceremony marking the tenth anniversary of the Jewish Ernst Ludwig Ehrlich Studienwerk on October 10, 2019, at the Jewish Museum Berlin.[1] Not because anti-Semitic crimes have increased in recent years and it was only a matter of time that this would lead to something extreme; or because the perceptions and consequently the assessments of those affected and the security authorities often diverge widely, and warnings are not always heard and responded to. Rather, the fundamental question arises as to the sense and benefit of anti-Semitism prevention if it is only reactive instead of proactive. Additional barriers and an increase in security personnel may suggest a sense of security, but in order for Jews to be able to live safely as Jews in Germany, there is a need for a proactive and thus publicly perceptible deconstruction of anti-Semitic prejudices, stereotypes, and narratives that can be encountered in a wide variety of contexts. And there is also a need for new perspectives on Jewish life in Germany, so that its public perception is not always reduced to anti-Semitism, the Shoah or the Middle East conflict. This is by no means to say that these are not aspects and facets of Jewish narratives - they are, although they can have quite different meanings or weightings for Jews individually.

---

[1] Siehe hierzu auch Jérôme Lombard, „Ort jüdischer Selbstbehauptung" (24.10.2019), https://www.juedische-allgemeine.de/unsere-woche/ort-juedischer-selbstbehauptung/?q=ELES (zuletzt abgerufen am 24.09.2021).

But the crucial difference is whether these aspects are defined in a foreign-determined way or are brought into discourses in a self-determined way.

Consequently, it must also be a matter of Jewish life becoming visible and experienceable in public in a different way. In a self-determined way. In recent years, numerous Jewish institutions, first and foremost the Central Council of Jews in Germany, the Central Welfare Organization of Jews in Germany (ZWSt) and the Ernst Ludwig Ehrlich Studienwerk (ELES), Jewish higher education institutions such as the Abraham Geiger College in Potsdam or the University of Jewish Studies in Heidelberg, but also civil Jewish interest groups, forums and platforms such as the Jewish Students Union Germany (JSUD), Hillel Deutschland e.V., Eruv Hub, Keshet e.V., Tamar e.V. or the magazine Jalta have contributed to this through their diverse work and commitment and have shown that Jewish life in Germany is not only a natural part of social plurality and diversity in Germany, but that this Jewish life itself is deeply plural and diverse. And that there are disputes and struggles - sometimes passionate and fierce - about what this can mean and what the limits of this diverse coexistence are. Perhaps this is what often causes irritation on the part of the rest of the population, because in view of a complex situation not everything seems comprehensible. But this Jewish complexity is exactly what a plural and open society must endure if it wants to define itself consistently as such and not leave it at mere rhetorical phrasing.

III.

Social plurality and diversity, however, is no longer something that can be perceived factually, but is increasingly determined by debates on identity politics. Through the radical diversity that some demand, others feel challenged; basically, one sees one's own self-image called into question by the position of the other. But does this necessarily have to be the case? Isn't it precisely a matter of being able to tolerate each other despite all the differences that exist, as long as one can agree to maintain social peace within the framework of *an agree-to-disagree?* Wouldn't it be important to explain to each other in a comprehensible way why the position of the other person causes such discomfort? What is one actually afraid of? Of progress or of regression, of continuity or of change?

But in the age of extremes 2.0 or 3.0, all forms of extreme attitudes and positions make themselves heard loudest and dominate social discourse with their bluster. In doing so, they make it quite 'easy' for themselves in the truest sense of the word, because that is precisely what the representatives of extreme positions are after all concerned with: reducing complexity, simplifications and polarizations instead of differentiations, ambivalences and dialectics. It certainly doesn't help that communication usually takes place in the echo chambers of social media, in which only one's own stance and positioning is brought to bear and clear friend-foe schemata are used. The interest is less in debate or discourse than in staking one's own claim to interpretive sovereignty, demanding it and asserting it. There seems to be less interest in negotiating compromises.

These identity-political debates and the way they are conducted also have an impact on the Jewish community in Germany, which is reflected not only in the recent debate about different Jewish self-understandings - halakhic or identity-related.[2] Here, too, attitudes and positions identified as left-wing and right-wing or progressive and conservative confront each other, not least because discourses on identity politics often overlap, regardless of whether they are about halakhah and religious practice, Israel, climate protection, the Bundestag elections, the withdrawal from Afghanistan, or gender issues. Or, indeed, about anti-Semitism and how to combat it. Debates and discourses are often multifactorial, also in the way they are conducted. In addition, there is also an intergenerational aspect, namely that the concept of community is conceived and

---

[2] Siehe hierzu exemplarisch das ZEIT-Doppelinterview mit Dr. Josef Schuster, Präsident des Zentralrats der Juden in Deutschland, und Dr. Meron Mendel, Leiter der Bildungsstätte Anne Frank „Wer ist Jude – und wer nicht?" (5.09.2021), https://www.zeit.de/kultur/2021-09/judentum-vaterjuden-identitaet-josef-schuster-meron-mendel-streitgespraech?utm_referrer=https%3A%2F%2Fwww.google.com%2F (zuletzt abgerufen am 24.09.2021).

understood less locally than globally in the sense of community. In other words, what constitutes a community has more to do with a voluntary network of like-minded people than with a kind of 'forced community' with the people one has locally. Which is not just about a selected aspect or understanding of identity, but about a connection of different identity markers.

One can certainly argue sociologically that this corresponds to generally observable phenomena and processes of increasing individualization, and that this thus poses challenges not only specifically to the Jewish community in Germany, but basically to most religious communities and social groups in the present. But in a relatively small community of just 250,000 people, of whom about 110,000 are organized through Jewish communities, this can also lead quite quickly to a fraying of community. This is one of the reasons why the Central Council of Jews in Germany, the Central Welfare Office of Jews in Germany and the Ernst Ludwig Ehrlich Studienwerk have made great efforts in recent years to create corresponding discourse spaces in which, despite all the existing diversity and even deviance, the question is asked as to what unites or can unite Jews. This question of common ground is the key to the vitality and resilience of the Jewish community in Germany. Both internally and externally.

IV.

But diversity is not only a characteristic of an open and pluralistic society. Because let's be honest, its enemies are no less diverse. Accordingly, anti-Semitism can also be articulated from extremely diverse attitudes and positioning. And this is precisely the central challenge for schools and other educational contexts. Since a differentiated and critical knowledge of the various manifestations of anti-Semitism cannot necessarily be assumed in these contexts, it is all the more important to network schools with the relevant competence centers and counseling centers. It is also important to create an awareness of the need to seek advice from these centers, especially when it is not really possible to understand how those affected experience discriminations. Being able to admit and acknowledge, like Stan Marsh from the U.S. television series South Park, "I get it now! I don't get it!".[1] This self-reflective insight is precisely what any form of education critical of anti-Semitism or racism should be about.

Some readers may wonder why this article links the issues of anti-Semitism and diversity. But in the aftermath of the Halle and Hanau attacks, there has been inflationary use of the Adornoian notion that an emancipated society is one in which one can "be different without fear."[2] If we are really serious about this, then this demand goes beyond ideologized particular interests and identity politics; it means not only emancipating ourselves, but also, in a sense, dialectically emancipating ourselves from ourselves. Being "Yourself different with(out) fear" opens up perspectives for us to live our diversities and differences, but in turn also takes us all into a shared responsibility for one another, no matter where we actually stand politically, religiously, socially, or identitarily. "Being different without fear" is a social vision we should strive for; and yet, I doubt that this very thing can simply be established as the status quo, as some think. Rather, what it means to "be different without fear" will have to be renegotiated over and over again as social conditions, frameworks and contexts change. This requires not least the courage to admit uncertainties and ambivalences and to endure different and conflicting needs and fears of loss; and the courage and willingness to moderate and dare to compromise. "Yourself different with(out) fear" also means a culture of remembrance in which it cannot be a matter of relativizing experiences and narratives or playing them off against each other on the basis of supposed victim competitions, but rather taking them seriously in their differences and their vulnerabilities. And to understand the perspectives they open up - and which are not least also perspectives on what people promise

---

[1] *South Park*, Season 11, Episode 1 "With Apologies to Jesse Jackson", https:// southpark.fandom.com/wiki/With_Apologies_to_Jesse_Jackson/Script (zuletzt abgerufen am 24.09.2021).

[2] Theodor W. Adorno, Minima Moralia, in: ders.: *Gesammelte Schriften*, Bd. 4. Frankfurt a.M. 1980, S. 114.

and hope for from society - as mosaic pieces of a possible common narrative. Even if it sounds exhausting and challenging, we need to come to an understanding about how we can tell the certainly not easy story of who we are as a plural society together, instead of fraying further and further into the juxtaposition that often seems easier and more comfortable.

I don't know if that can be an effective way to combat anti-Semitism. But I also don't believe that anti-Semitism can be combated solely with increased security precautions or with the establishment of state or federal offices for anti-Semitism officers, especially if the latter are only capable of acting symbolically due to a lack of resources. An anti-Semitism-free society requires something much more fundamental than that or merely making Jewish visible in public discourse. It is the *dispositif* of the discourse that needs to change. Which we need to change. Because I honestly don't want to celebrate the coming Yom Kippur with a feeling of latent threat, nor do I want to ask myself during the next conflict between Israel and Hamas and the anti-Semitic hatred that is unleashed on social media, but also in physical violence, what is still actually keeping me in Germany ...

If, in the end, it is merely a matter of a colorful Jewish visibility suitable for Instagram, instead of changing something socially fundamental and sustainable with regard to perceptions and perspectives on Judaism in Germany, then, to be honest, we might as well save the celebratory year 1700 and all the anniversaries that may follow it. Because it is not always about the spotlight in the negative as well as in the positive sense. Jews in Germany also have a right to something like normality. However boring or spectacular this may turn out to be should be left up to them.

P. S.: But hey, "maybe I'm wrong, but I want to believe in humanity," as Carole King once sang. For our sake, I hope she's not.

Chapter Six

Judeophobia 2.0 as a Cultural Tradition of Educated Elites: Current Anti-Semitism and the Echoes of the Past

Monika Schwarz-Friesel

Introduction

Not only since the attack on the synagogue in Halle, not only in the course of the Corona pandemic with its rampant anti-Semitic conspiracy fantasies on the net, not only in the recent anti-Israel demonstrations on the streets of German cities, hostility towards Jews has again taken on fearsome proportions 75 years after the Auschwitz experience: Although empirical research on anti-Semitism has been warning for more than ten years that the taboo on anti-Semitic statements is also eroding in the middle of society and that anti-Jewish ideas are being communicated more audibly and confidently, in the fight against anti-Semitism in politics, the media and the public, the causal relationship between the educated middle and the social fringes is often misinterpreted, as reflected in headlines such as "Anti-Semitism has reached the middle." In fact, however, historically, anti-Jewish ideas always came from the center, from the writings of the learned and educated, before they reached the street. For hatred of Jews is not primarily a social-psychological but a cultural phenomenon, and Judeophobic topoi are an integral part of Western religious and intellectual history. Accordingly, it must be repeatedly stated that concepts and patterns of language hostile to Jews have been firmly and deeply anchored in cultural memory for 2,000 years, precisely because art and culture, because not only the uneducated marginal figures, but also the masterminds who shaped the cultural sphere of society, have passed them on over the centuries.[1] This tradition, as the ongoing debate about the anti-Israel statements of the post-colonial scholar Achille Mbembe shows, is not only unbroken today, but has reached an extent of Holocaust relativization, denial of Israel-hatred as anti-Semitism, and a rejection of memory culture that has not been seen since the *Historikerstreit*.

This article compressively outlines some of the findings on the prevalence of Jew-hatred on the Internet 2.0 and then highlights the parallels as well as the connections between classical hostility toward Jews and current manifestations of educated debates on anti-Semitism.

No Purification: Anti-Jewish Resentment and its Unbroken Continuity in the World Wide Web 2.0

The Internet represents the most important communication space today. Due to the specifics of Internet communication, such as active network participation, speed, free accessibility, multimodality, anonymity, global interconnection, and the increasing relevance of social media as an opinion-forming source of information in society as a whole, the rapid, unfiltered, and almost limitless dissemination of anti-Jewish ideas has reached an extent, in purely quantitative terms alone, that has never been seen before in history. The digitalization of information and communication technology has made "anti-Semitism 2.0" multipliable online in a fast, multi-modal, diffuse and recipient-unspecific way. Every day, thousands of new

---

[1] In the long history of anti-Judaism, church fathers and priests were often the only ones who could read and write at all and who articulated anti-Jewish ideas in their writings and sermons. By no means was and is hostility to Jews a problem of poorly educated people, as can often be read. But the debates about the journalist Jakob Augstein and the anti-Israel poem by Günter Grass have already shown that many in our society still cling to the narrow, false image of the 'stupid Springer-boot anti-Semite'. Education does not protect against anti-Jewish resentment. In the USA, for example, so-called campus anti-Semitism has been taking on explosive proportions at elite universities for years. See, among others, Monika Schwarz-Friesel, „Antisemitismus an Universitäten: die lange Tradition gebildeter Judenfeindschaft," in: *Gender, Politik, Universität. Gegen Diskriminierung an Hochschulen*, 2016, 1, TU Berlin: Die Zentrale Frauenbeauftragte, S. 22–23, http://www.audiatur-online.ch/2016/06/16/antisemitismus-an-universitaeten-die-lange-tradition-gebildeter-judenfeindschaft/.

anti-Semitisms are posted, adding to the anti-Jewish texts, images, and videos that have been stored and viewable online for years. In a ten-year comparison, the number of anti-Semitic online comments has tripled in some cases between 2007 and 2018. Moreover, there is hardly any area of discourse in Web 2.0 where users do not run the risk of encountering anti-Semitic texts, even if they do not actively search for them. The Internet acts as a multiplier, especially in the everyday communication areas of social media, because it makes anti-Semitisms accessible on a large scale, spreads them on all levels of Web 2.0, and thus encourages the normalization of Jew-hatred. Analyses of Google searches and advice portals show that often with just one click after entering a keyword such as Jew(s), Judaism, Passover or Israel, users are unprepared to encounter anti-Semitisms. In some cases, these remain undeleted for years, e.g. the question "Why are Jews always so evil?" at Gutefrage.net, which has been viewable since 2011. Anti-Semitisms are thus by no means found only in politically oriented or radical areas of discourse, but above all in the much-used everyday media of the Web. Corpus studies on comments regarding solidarity actions against anti-Semitism ("Nie wieder Judenhass" and "Berlin trägt Kippa") also demonstrate the infiltration of these communication structures, with over 37 percent anti-Semitisms in some cases. Global links and multimodal linking on the Web play a special role in the transmission of anti-Semitism. That users receive indoctrination instead of information and discussion is evident in all major social media, e.g., Twitter, YouTube, Facebook, and also in entertainment websites as diverse as fan forums, blogs, and online bookstores.

Current manifestations of anti-Semitism in the 21st century are cognitively based on traditional stereotypes, some of which are ancient, and emotionally based on the collective emotional value of hatred, and thus represent a modern reactivation of culturally embedded resentment. Israel-related anti-Semitism, a dominant manifestation of current hostility toward Jews on Web 2.0, follows the age-old adaptation pattern of Jew-hatred of focusing negatively on that form of existence of Judaism - in this case the state of Israel - that can be opportunely defamed.

The echo of the past is particularly clear on the Internet: The old anti-Judaism with its destructive semantics is still deeply embedded in communicative memory: Classic stereotypes of hostility toward Jews are a major feature of anti-Semitism 2.0, accounting for over 54.02 percent. It should be noted that Jew-hatred and Israel-hatred form a conceptual symbiosis that is determined to a large extent by the collective concept of the "Eternal Jew" with its characteristics, constructed over centuries, of "Jews as foreigners/others/evil, as usurers, exploiters and money men, as vengeful schemers and power seekers, murderers, ritual and blood cult practitioners, land robbers, destroyers and conspirators. Apart from superficial variations, there are no significant differences between the anti-Semitisms of right-wing, left-wing, Muslim, and centrist users. The writers refer to classical stereotypes of hostility towards Jews and use homogeneous Judeophobic arguments, which are altogether determined by an emotional attitude (see Trachtenberg on the forms of demonization in the Middle Ages). Through the language use patterns of demarcation and devaluation, stereotypes hostile to Jews are constantly reproduced and thus remain in the collective consciousness. Even the experience of the Holocaust has not broken this tradition. Moreover, numerous strategies of defense, denial, reinterpretation, and marginalization of society's hatred of Jews are evident. The ostentatious anti-Semitisms are thereby reclassified in pseudo-political discourse as "criticism of Israel" and, for example, in German-language rap as "freedom of art or opinion" in order to appear politically correct and socially appropriate in accordance with the official assessment in post-Holocaust consciousness.

Accordingly, anti-Semitisms are often coded in a camouflaged way: Not the lexemes "Jews" and "Judaism," but substitutions such as "Israelis," "Zionism," ciphers such as "Rothschild," vague paraphrases such as "those influential circles," or rhetorical questions such as "Why do Zionists act as criminals?" are used to disseminate anti-Jewish semantics. The increase in the articulation of Nazi comparisons, brute pejoratives - "filth, plague, cancer" - and violent fantasies in the sense of eliminatory anti-Semitism, however, also proves the tendency of verbal radicalization as well as a significant lowering of the taboo threshold. The conclusion after six years of extensive research is therefore: Jew-hatred is omnipresent in Web 2.0 and already habitualized to a large extent (see in detail Schwarz-Friesel 2019a and b).

Voices from the Educated Middle: Anti-Semitism Denial and the Perception and Acceptance Problem.

But it is not only in the digital space that we see such tendencies. Triggered by the debate surrounding Mbembe's anti-Israel remarks, an ongoing debate has developed since 2020 in the commentary and article sections of the mainstream media as well as the social media of the Internet around colonial history, memory culture, and the internationally recognized IHRA definition of anti-Semitism. Under euphonious names such as "cosmopolitanism," "liberal culture of remembrance," and "enlightenment and freedom of expression," academically established individuals spread attention-seeking and always media-staged appeals that trivialize the civilizational rupture of the Shoah, deny the dominant variant of Israel-related anti-Semitism, and favor false or overly narrow definitions of Jew-hatred (e.g., as racism or xenophobia) (see also Friesel 2021).

Instead of following the rampant anti-Semitic demonstrations on the occasion of Gaza 2014 and Gaza 2021 as well as the annual anti-Israel events on Al Kuds Day, the Halle attack, and the statistics on rising anti-Semitic crime (especially in symbiosis Jew-Israel hatred; cf. In the wake of the Berlin Senate's 2020 anti-Semitism report, which unanimously condemns Judeophobic statements in the camouflage garb of "criticism of Israel," instead of showing scholars who demonize the Jewish state with crude analogies and topoi of anti-Semitism clear limits for their irresponsibility in dealing with such language structures, voices are increasingly and vociferously rising to defend, even approve of, this rhetoric. Added to this are the now obligatory petitions to reinforce "freedom of speech" and legitimize unambiguously anti-Israel movements like BDS. In the case of Mbembe, 700 African artists and intellectuals wrote a letter to Angela

Merkel convincing her that these were all "lying accusations" and that Mbembe's critics only came from the right-wing.[2] This was followed by signatures of German and internationally active persons from the academic milieu, who - pleading for "cosmopolitanism" - criticized the decision of the German government not to give any more support to the anti-Semitic BDS (which ultimately pursues the goal of making the Jewish state of Israel disappear) as well as a plea for a "new definition of anti-Semitism" (see critically Bernstein et al. 2021).

The fact that even 10,000 signatures cannot deny the fact that Mbembe has irresponsibly written texts with classical topoi of hostility to Jews is ignored. All public debates on anti-Semitism in recent years (e.g. those on Günther Grass and Jacob Augstein) have shown that parts of German society have a massive perception and acceptance problem regarding the reality and extent of current hostility towards Jews. Contrary to all findings from historical and current research, anti-Semitism is seen almost exclusively as a right-wing phenomenon by uneducated or backward-looking, anti-democratic and nationalistically oriented individuals. This inadmissibly narrows the broad spectrum of anti-Jewish resentment, levels its anchoring in society as a whole and, in particular, its cultural foundation in the educational canon of the Occident. The Mbembe case revealed a degree of ignorance, suppression, reinterpretation and double standards that had never been seen before on this subject. And it reveals the tip of an iceberg: Hatred of Jews is currently manifesting itself not only in Web 2.0, more openly and unabashedly than ever before - as what it always was and is: as resentment directed against Jewish existence in the world.[3] Accordingly - not only since Corona - conspiracy and annihilation fantasies flood the worldwide web

---

[2] https://simoninou.files.wordpress.com/2020/05/brief-von-afrikanischen_ intellektuellen_an-die-dt-bundeskanzlerin_-angela-merkel.pdf.

[3] Monika Schwarz-Friesel, *Judenhass im Internet. Antisemitismus als kulturelle Konstante und kollektives Gefühl*, Berlin 2019.

every minute: "Israel bred Corona", "Destroy Israel!", "Death to Zionism", "Death to Israel", "Free Palestine".[4]

The ancient concept of 'Jews as evil par excellence' thus finds its modern expressions (S. Schwarz-Friesel 2019a, b).

The Israelization of Anti-Semitic Semantics

No less explosive, if not even more alarming, than the hate-filled net expressions are voices from the cultural and academic establishment that deny, trivialize, or reinterpret the dominant variant of current Jew-hatred, of all things, Israel-related anti-Semitism.[5] This has demonstrably been particularly pronounced for years. In research, we have therefore long spoken of an "Israelization of anti-Semitism": anti-Jewish stereotypes are projected onto the Jewish state, the most important symbol of Jewish life in the world, and hatred of Israel becomes the link for all varieties of hostility toward Jews. But the "renowned", "well-known", "award-winning" comedians, writers, musicians and academics as well as journalists in the post-Holocaust society do not want to be called "anti-Semites".

Instead, criticism and debunking of anti-Semitic statements is inevitably followed by the accused's routine declaration that they are "appalled," "dismayed," even "stunned" by the accusation of

---

[4] "Free Palestine!" is in many contexts a cipher for the call to make Israel disappear from the map, and is based on the slogan "From the river to the sea, Palestine will be free!" For many years, such ciphers have been an integral part of anti-Semitic detour communication, which uses camouflage techniques to formally de-radicalize radical content (on this, see, among others, Lars Rensmann, "Zion als Chiffre," in: Monika Schwarz-Friesel (ed.), *Gebildeter Antisemitismus*, Baden-Baden 2015, S. 93–116).

[5] Vgl. etwa Moshe Zuckermann in conversation with Johannes Nichelmann: https://www.deutschlandfunkkultur.de/moshe-zuckermann-zur-debatte-um-mbembe-antizionismus.1013.de.html?dram:article_id=475490 sowie Micha Brumlik im Gespräch mit Tanya Lieske: https://www.deutschlandfunk.de/solidaritaetsbrief-fuer-achille-mbembe-vergleich-bedeutet.691.de.html?dram:article_id=475977. Siehe hierzu auch Evyatar Friesel, „Die umgedrehten ideologischen Pyramiden der anti-zionistischen Juden: Das Fallbeispiel Moshe Zuckermann", https://www.audiatur-online.ch/2017/04/18/die-umgedrehten-ideologischen-pyramiden-der-anti-zionistischen-juden-das-fallbeispiel-moshe-zuckermann/.

anti-Semitism. These defensive strategies have been extensively researched as an integral part of the anti-Semitism denial discourse.[6] To play with linguistic structures against the better knowledge of the danger of rhetoric and its persuasive effect is stylized as freedom of speech. With astonishing ignorance, the same arguments are reproduced and thrown into the public discourse, even by intellectuals and people with academic degrees, without any factual basis, assigned solely to the surreal enemy image ISRAEL, without taking into account empirical data or expert findings[7]: "Criticism of Israel" is subject to a taboo (this is not to be stated in reality), political criticism is not to be equated with hatred of Jews (as if any seriously arguing person ever claimed this), and in the end it is difficult to clearly distinguish anti-Semitism from criticism of Israel (although research has long since presented analytical criteria and deciphering categories for a precise distinction[8]).

---

[6] See here Monika Schwarz-Friesel/Jehuda Reinharz, *Die Sprache der Judenfeindschaft im 21. Jahrhundert*, Berlin/Boston 2013, Kap. 11, https://www.degruyter.com/view/title/123466?rskey=D5BOTK&result=36.

[7] Representative and typical of such lay voices, see for example Yossi Bartal in conversation with Inge Günther on June 24, 2019 in the Frankfurter Rundschau: "I experience the climate in Germany, especially after the Bundestag resolution on the boycott movement BDS, in such a way that any fundamental criticism of the conditions in Israel/Palestine is excluded or even criminalized." A "free discourse" is being "stifled," https://www.fr.de/kultur/interview-yossi-bartal-juedisches-museum-berlin-12665805.html. Reality gives the lie to this statement, because by no means is serious criticism of Israeli actions, which is often and sharply formulated in the media and politics, "criminalized" as anti-Semitism. Hardly any debate is conducted as freely and intensively as that on the Middle East conflict. Cf: https://www.zeit.de/politik/deutschland/2014-08/israel-medien-kritik. An empirical study has also proven that the much-vaunted taboo of criticism does not exist (Monika Schwarz-Friesel 2019, Judenhass im Internet, S. 135ff.).

[8] Cf. Monika Schwarz-Friesel/Jehuda Reinharz, *Die Sprache der Judenfeindschaft*, Kap. 3–5 sowie Armin Lange/Kerstin Mayerhofer/Dina Porat/Lawrence H. Schiffman (Hg.), *Comprehending and Confronting Antisemitism. A Multi-Faceted Approach*, https://www.degruyter.com/view/title/547255.

But for many artists and academics it seems inconceivable that anti-Semitic ideas could come from the mouths of educated, enlightened and liberal-minded people. "Witch hunt", "lynching", "oppression", "McCarthyism"[9]- with such brute vocabulary academics support Mbembe without expertise, without checking what the really relevant research has to say.[10] The latter distinguishes for good reason between verbal anti-Semitism (i.e. the forms of expression) and conceptual anti-Semitism (the attitude): An anti-Semitic expression always has an effect, also and especially unconsciously, through its semantics; it always carries stereotypes and clichés into society, regardless of who expresses it and whether it is articulated in an intentional or non-intentional anti-Semitic way.[11] Even education and an Enlightenment attitude do not automatically prevent the production of anti-Semitic speech patterns; the entire history of the Occident shows this. Voltaire, Fichte, Hegel, Dickens and many others were liberal-minded writers and scholars, but their works contain verbally explicit demonizations of Jews. In the end, the heated Mbembe debate was about precisely this aspect, but it was completely lost in the highly emotional discussions. Since we know about the potential of anti-Semitic rhetoric to influence the collective consciousness, we should, indeed must - if we seriously want to combat anti-Semitism in society as a whole - in principle always criticize and reject as such statements that encode Judeophobic topoi and combine explosive catchwords, regardless of the person and their education or attitude.

---

[9] See, among others, the historian Andreas Eckert: https://www.swr.de/swr2/leben-und-gesellschaft/antisemitismus-vorwuerfe-gegen-achille-mbembe-anzeichen-einer-hexenjagd-104.html as well as the pedagogue Micha Brumlik on 3sat: https://www.3sat.de/kultur/kulturzeit/der-fall-mbembe-100.html.

[10] See, among other things, the references, literature references and analyses at https://www.stopantisemitismus.de/.

[11] See, among others, Monika Schwarz-Friesel, *Sprache und Emotion*, Tübingen 2013, Kap. 11, and Richard A. Friedmann, *The Neuroscience of Hate Speech*, 2018, https://www.nytimes.com/2018/10/31/opinion/caravan-hate-speech-bowers-sayoc.html.

Public Debates on Anti-Semitism and Lay Culture: Misconceptualizations and Reinterpretations

The majority of academics from philologies outside of anti-Semitism research, as well as publicists and artists, marginalize or completely brush aside this crucial aspect. On the topic of "modern Jew-hatred" they have neither basic research nor empirical studies to show, but opinions presented with much emotionality. But opinions are no substitute for valid research results, which, for example, are the result of years of quantitative and qualitative text analysis. A well-known problem becomes apparent here: lay communication[12] has long characterized public debates on anti-Semitism, with denial and reinterpretation of Israel-related anti-Semitisms being typical. In the current case, one likes to pull this platitude out of the drawer: comparing is legitimate in science and does not mean equating. Yes, if only they were factually based, appropriate comparisons and not fantasy constructs with slogans of anti-Jewish rhetoric! Conceptualizing Israel as a Nazi, racist or apartheid state follows the principle of de-realization, interpreting Jewish life from the point of view of Jew-haters - phantasms devoid of any reality.

In the recent debate about texts by the colonial scholar Achille Mbembe, which with surreal analogies and emotional superlatives display characteristics of just such patterns of language use, this imbalance comes to the fore with a force that should shake up politics, the media, and civil society. But it does not. No gain in knowledge can be observed. It is not facts but feelings that determine this discourse, which has become a battle for interpretive sovereignty. In many places, the media and the public reinforce this impression: instead of using expert and research categories, they

---

[12] Imagine discussing with citizens, journalists and politicians the possibilities of therapy for tumor cells in the brain without inviting brain researchers and physicians who specialize in this field. Nobody would take such activities too seriously. However, this is exactly what happens almost every week on the topic of anti-Semitism: publicists, journalists, activists tune in to the media and give advice, discuss possible reasons and consequences. Cf. also the editorial in the Jüdische Allgemeine of 29.11.2018: https://www.juedische-allgemeine.de/politik/die-floskelkultur/.

give a voice to anyone who raises it particularly loudly. Without any critical reference, they print comments by educated laymen, e.g. on "anti-Semitism as a general misanthropy", which is simply wrong, or on the IHRA definition of anti-Semitism, which was developed by internationally renowned researchers.[13] However, anti-Semitism is not general misanthropy, but exclusively hostility towards Jews. Jews are hated and stigmatized as Jews and not as a minority.[14]

Anti-Semitism also has little in common with xenophobia and general discrimination, because Jews were and are not 'strangers' in their respective countries, but integrated citizens for 200 years, who gave and give no cause for fear. Jew-hatred is also by no means linked to an anti-modern and backward-looking worldview, but can be found among left-wing progressives who speak out for multiculturalism and against nationalism, who stand up for modern enlightenment and equal rights in a forward-looking way, but at the same time indulge in a Jewophobic hatred of Israel in the "name of humanism". In this respect, hatred of Jews is not to be equated with racism (although precisely this equation is articulated particularly frequently in public discourse), but can also be found among liberal, educated and anti-racist-minded people. Their tolerance extends to all minorities and idiosyncrasies, except the Jewish state.

Jew-hatred in the variant of Israel-hatred is the dominant variant of modern anti-Semitism in the 21st century and at the same time the least combated. Explanations that attribute Israel-related anti-Semitism monocausally to the Middle East conflict fail to recognize the true character of this form of manifestation. Hatred of Israel continues the long cultural tradition of projection and is typically an expression of opportune conformity. Yet debates invariably drift away from this

---

[13] See, for example, Peter Ullrich's expert opinion on the IHRA definition: https://www. rosalux.de/publikation/id/41168/gutachten-zur-arbeitsdefinition-antisemitismus-der-ihra and the clear rejection by anti-Semitism research: https://www.tu-berlin.de/fileadmin/i65/Veranstaltungen/2019/Stellungnahme_Wetzel.pdf.

[14] Jews are not seen by anti-Semites as a minority, but as 'THE others'. This has the status of an epistemic category. Jews are the counter-design to one's own form of existence, which is to be rejected and negated not only in parts, but absolutely and absolutely. See also Monika Schwarz-Friesel, Judenhass im Internet, pp. 33ff. and 144ff.

realization. How simple and effective it would be for someone who articulates anti-Semitic topoi to regret the explosive verbal slippage in his rhetoric. In the Mbembe case, however, he vehemently and irrationally cast himself as a victim of "German racism. He discredited the FDP politician Lorenz Deutsch with vague insinuations that the latter might have contact with the neo-Nazi scene and insinuated the "diabolical idea" of an "anti-Semitic Negro.[15] He demanded an apology "until my last breath"[16] from the anti-Semitism commissioner Felix Klein, who had rightly criticized Mbembe's text passages with reference to valid research findings. In this absurd theater, which makes every anti-Semitism expert stop laughing, there was only one person who should have apologized as soon as possible for the accumulation of verbal slips: Mbembe himself.

But this regret, which presupposes the insight of having used a dangerous and inadequate rhetoric, did not come. After his self-justification discourse (which did not take factuality too seriously, as was already revealed in the *FAZ*[17]), he went into the perpetrator-victim reversal with tearfulness in the "Gigantische[n] Defamierungskampagne". He did not retract his anti-Israel statements. Does the "well-known and renowned scientist from Cameroon[18]" not know about the danger of certain speech patterns? Does he have to call people whose view he does not accept "Pharisees" and "Zealots"[19] of all things (terms that were used for centuries as swear words for Jews) and use the catchword "an eye for an eye, a tooth for a tooth," which is used inflationarily in anti-Semitic discourse? Does he really have to accuse the Jewish state

---

[15] https://taz.de/Mbembe-zum-Antisemitismusvorwurf/!5684094/.

[16] Ebd.

[17] Jürgen Kaube, "Who Lynched Achille Mbembe?", 10.05.2020, https://www.faz.net/aktuell/feuilleton/debatten/antisemitismus-debatte-um-den-philosoph-achille-mbembe-16761907.html.

[18] Alan Posener, "Jörg Häntzschel or the Incapacity for Self-Criticism" 29.04.2020, https://starke-meinungen.de/blog/2020/04/29/joerg-haentzschel-oder-die-unfaehigkeit-zur-selbstkritik/.

[19] Gerald Beyrodt, "Anti-Semites Are Still the Others," 01.05.2020, https://www.deutschlandfunkkultur.de/zur-causa-mbembe-antisemiten-sind-immer-noch-die-anderen.1079.de.html?dram:article_id=475841.

of apartheid "worse than in South Africa," accuse it of "fanatical extermination," call for its "worldwide isolation," and de-realize the "occupation of Palestine" as the "greatest moral scandal of our time"?[20] Crude superlatives and explosive metaphors in the ductus of populism that Mbembe spreads; not a trace of serious scholarship and the benefit of doubt in his own point of view. How beneficial and enlightening in the best sense it would have been if Mbembe had shown insight and publicly admitted to using inappropriate and dangerous, historically toxic language and rhetoric. How much this would have advanced the work of combating anti-Semitism. But the self-righteous insistence without any critical self-doubt and the perpetrator-victim reversal with respect to critics characterized the behavior of the post-colonial scholar (and his adepts).

Double standards and double standards: the hubris of moralists

Let us now imagine the following scenario: Exactly the same statements would not have been published by the scholar of colonialism Mbembe, but by the AfD man Björn Höcke.[21] How different the reactions would have been? A pronounced double standard with regard to right-wing and left-wing hostility toward

---

[20] Cf. Mbembe in the preface of the book *Apartheid Israel: The Politics of an Analogy*, 2015.

[21] Such hypothetical re-framings, i.e., the re-contextualization of per se problematic statements, generally help to reflect on double standards in the evaluation of verbal anti-Semitisms and to sensitize to the fact that it is the statement alone that is explosive, not (necessarily) the person. This was also the case in the debate about the anti-Israel poem by Günter Grass, after all a winner of the Nobel Prize for Literature. (See on this: Monika Schwarz-Friesel in conversation with Klaus Pokatzky, 10.04.2012, https://www.deutschlandfunkkultur.de/dieser-text-bedient-moderne-antisemitische-klischees.954.de.html?dram:article_id=147146). Verbal anti-Semitisms have a stigmatizing and stereotype-consolidating potential qua semantics. Solely the meaning content is relevant, not the person and his intention, not his social position or ethnicity, not the context. For human cognition processes language autonomously, i.e. independently of speaker intention and functionality (see fn. 11). By the way, this also applies to verbal racisms: Language-sensitive people therefore do not use loaded words such as the N-word, because these automatically and uncontrollably trigger discriminatory connotations and associations.

Israel becomes transparent. We have long been familiar with this from the debates about BDS: declaring "war" on neo-Nazis and right-wing radicals, but eyes wide shut in the face of left-wing anti-Zionism and anti-Israelism. This is not the way to fight anti-Semitism in society as a whole. As long as there are double standards of evaluation for the spread of (verbal) anti-Semitism, any work against hostility towards Jews will remain ineffective. Together with the usual outrage staging such as "the discussion about Israel-related anti-Semitism" harms the "urgent fight against real anti-Semitism", one is engaged in a "character assassination campaign", and one draws on a "misuse of the term anti-Semitism", this time, however, moralizing is taken to the extreme.[22] Here a "new German self-confidence" appears, which Jews as well as the state of Israel can and would like to do without. As one reads in the *Frankfurter Rundschau*[23]: "Aleida Assmann has aptly named the conflict situation at this point: 'Now a dividing line runs between those who are anxious to support and improve the state of Israel with their criticism, and those who are determined to immunize it against any criticism [...]'"[24]. Is it "accurate" for Germans to presume to "seek to improve" the Jewish state with a raised index finger?

Anyone who knows only a fraction about the past and the history of Jew-hatred should feel uneasy at such statements. Such hubris could only develop because of the illusion in Germany of an enlightened post-Holocaust society that has learned from the horrors of history and has emerged purified. This "purification process," however, never took place across the board. For, as historical and discourse-analytical research of the past 30 years has documented in detail, there was no real coming to terms with the past after 1945, no serious

---

[22] See, among others. https://www.openpetition.de/petition/blog/einspruch-gegen-sprachregelungen-fuer-hochschulen.

[23] https://www.fr.de/kultur/gesellschaft/missbraeuchlicheindienstnahme-13751102.html.

[24] The quotation comes from an article in the Frankfurter Rundschau, in which Assmann calls the critical commentary on Mbembe's anti-Israeli and anti-Semitic rhetoric "denunciation" and makes "proposals for a definition of anti-Semitism" without addressing the relevant expert research: https://www.fr.de/kultur/gesellschaft/klima-verdachts-verunsicherung-denunziation-13749410.html.

discussion of guilt and shame. Rather, perpetrator-victim reversals and a collective defense against guilt developed with the concept of innocent perpetrators. Building on this, a know-it-all mentality has emerged among left-wing and right-wing intellectuals in recent years that is disturbing. As if in a kind of missionary urge, these moralists, who declare themselves to be humanists, enlightened and responsible citizens, speak out against Jews and Israelis from an elevated pedestal, as can be seen not only in the public statements but also in the many letters from academics to the Central Council of Jews in Germany and the Israeli Embassy in Berlin, which include names, addresses and numerous self-disclosures.[25] The 'Holocaust experience' is not used as an ethical or emotional guideline for shame and humility, but rather as a legitimation value for a special, exaggerated self-confidence towards the descendants of the victims. Like head teachers to underage children who have allegedly learned nothing from history (this is all too often the collective reproach), they appear to Jewish citizens and Israelis, give advice, punitive sermons, make suggestions about how Israel should be shaped and the conflict resolved, and how the Central Council should behave.

This hubris is the result of the sham reappraisal of the Holocaust, the cherished and sometimes gleefully celebrated illusion of perfect purification and overcoming guilt. Restraint in criticism of Israel because of the German past? A "catechism" of remembrance culture forcing Germans into a Procrustean bed, as an Australian colonial researcher named Moses may claim in the German quality media in 2021? The opposite is the case. From Germany's specific historical responsibility, a universal claim - a kind of global ethic, as it were - has been derived for the present and the future to speak out against all injustice and discrimination from now on. The fact that in the end this virtue guard mentality is primarily and often uniquely directed at Israel and the Middle East conflict is not reflected. From the mantra that one has "learned the lessons" and would "never again remain silent in the face of suffering and oppression," these individuals demand that German Jews and Israelis "finally show insight" and

---

[25] Siehe hierzu ausführlich das Kapitel „Judenfeindschaft als Missionarsdrang" in Monika Schwarz-Friesel/Jehuda Reinharz, *Die Sprache der Judenfeindschaft*, S. 323ff.

"exercise humanity,[26]" thus imputing cognitive and emotional deficits to them in principle. The "height of the fall" is intensified by the unfortunate experience of the Jewish people: Not even the Holocaust could turn Jews into "people of moral integrity who sympathize with the Palestinians.[27]" A victim-perpetrator reversal expressed with great self-satisfaction can hardly be codified more clearly. The fact that the argumentation of these moralists is based on deep anti-Judaic thought patterns makes the whole argument absurd. It shows that nothing has been learned from history: Using classic Judeophobic and anti-Jewish rhetoric rather exposes the absence of the purification so often invoked.

For advice on how Jews should behave, how they should live, how they should conform to "good Christian people" has a long tradition in the history of Western hostility toward Jews. Even the explicitly well-meaning thinkers and politicians committed to the Enlightenment who advocated the 'good' and the 'emancipation' of the Jewish population (such as Abbé Grégoire and Wilhelm von Dohm in the late 18th century) could not accept 'Jewishness' as it was and demanded assimilation to the "good Christian people." No one has captured this primal core of anti-Jewish resentment as aptly as Léon Poliakov in his book Bréviaire de la haine (1951) on the motive of the 'Final Solution': that Jews were killed simply because they were Jews. No social envy, no economic or social reasons led to the catastrophe, as is often claimed - distorting the reason for the Shoah - but the centuries-old hatred of occidental anti-Judaism. The uniquely monstrous: to exterminate Jews for the good of mankind (so Himmler in his speeches). Exactly this demand is found today in relation to Israel: radically as a demand for the dissolution of the Jewish state or camouflagingly well-meaning as "change in the name of humanity." Where are these "humanistic" voices when it

---

[26] Hunderte von E-Mails enthalten diese Floskeln; siehe Monika Schwarz-Friesel/ Jehuda Reinharz, Die Sprache der Judenfeindschaft, S. 328ff. und S. 369.

[27] The contrast between 'good and bad Jews' that is often expressed in this context is striking: Good Jews are those murdered in the Holocaust or those who condemn Israel, 'bad Jews' are those who like to live in Israel and those who defend Israel (see ibid., p. 376ff.).

comes to the real hot spots and problems of world politics: around ISIS, Syria, Russia, Turkey or China, around Poland and Hungary, just to name a few? There, opinion-suppressing and anti-democratic processes are underway. But the unique and highly emotional focus, it is on Israel, a stable democracy.[28]

These voices, precisely because they come from the educated elite, hinder the effective fight against the strengthening Jew-hatred in a particularly damaging way, because they are not immediately met with the suspicion of tumid Jew-hatred like right-wing radicals or populists (who - nota bene - demand exactly the same thing), because many in society listen to them, one nods and secretly says to oneself highly satisfied: "Yes, this evil Israel, why should it be sacrosanct, they are no better than the Nazis back then" - and thus one is at the concept of the collective Jew and in the heart of anti-Semitic thinking and feeling. This is how extremists, radicals, fundamentalists and populists get support. The right-wing extremist poster texts such as "Israel is our misfortune!"

Conclusion

Classical hostility toward Jews is by no means in retreat or hardly to be found in current communication (as can be read or heard more often lately) - the stereotypes and the intense feelings on which anti-Semitic resentment has been based for centuries continue to have an unbroken effect. The chameleon anti-Semitism changes only its external manifestations over time, but its content remains. On the Internet, a virulent hatred of Jews is articulated on a daily basis,

---

[28] Israeli policy is much and sharply criticized. The Jewish state is not sacrosanct. As in any other country in the world, there are injustices, corruption, police violence, discrimination, controversial state actions, nationalist decisions, treaty violations in Israel. All of this is reported (not least by the Israeli press itself). It is not that criticism is made, but how it is argumentatively justified and linguistically formulated that is crucial to this discussion. Serious critics, of whom there are many, do not resort to Nazi comparisons and Judeophobic topoi, nor do they use the communicative initiative strategy of defense and denial such as "I am not an anti-Semite, but ..." as a preventive measure to protect themselves from accusations of anti-Semitism. Legitimate criticism does not need such justification.

projecting the traditional medieval stereotypes onto Israel in constant repetition. The hatred of Israel displays all the characteristics of the old reactivated hatred of Jews and shows the continuity and adaptability of this cultural category. In the feature discussions and signature campaigns with statements deligitimizing Israel, these radical voices receive support and resonance from the educated center. In the last two decades, many academics have not only not learned anything from the debates and research on current Jew-hatred, they are even taking a fatal step backwards with regard to the urgently required educational efforts.

Bibliography

Audit of Anti-Semitic Incidents, ADL Report 2018.

Antisemitismus in verfassungsfeindlichen Ideologien und Bestrebungen. Broschüre der Berliner Senatsverwaltung. Berlin, Juni 2020. Online unter: https://www.berlin.de/sen/inneres/verfassungsschutz/publikationen/info/

Bernstein, J., 2020. *Antisemitismus an Schulen in Deutschland. Befunde – Analysen – Handlungsoptionen*. Weinheim: Beltz Juventa.

Bernstein, J./Rensmann, L./Schwarz-Friesel, M., 2021. *Faktisch falsche Prämissen*. Online unter: https://www.juedische-allgemeine. de/politik/faktisch-falsche-praemissen/.

Friesel, E., 2011. "On the complexities of modern Jewish identity: Contemporary Jews against Israel", *Israel Affairs*, Vol. 17, No. 4, October 2011, 504–519.

Friesel, E., 2021. *"Antisemitism-Lite" in Contemporary Germany*. Besa-Center: https://besacenter.org/antisemitism-germany-today/.

Kantor Centre Report 2018. University of Tel Aviv.

Lange, A. et al, 2020. *Comprehending and Confronting Antisemitism.* Boston: de Gruyter. Open access: https://www.degruyter. com/view/title/547255

Nirenberg, D., 2013. Anti-Judaism. The Western Tradition. New York: W. W. Norton & Company.

Poliakov, L., 1956. *Harvest of hate*. London.

Recherche und Informationsstelle Antisemitismus Berlin (RIAS), 2017. Antisemitische Vorfälle 2017. Berlin. Online unter: https:// report-antisemitism.de/media/bericht-antisemitischer-vorfaelle-2017.pdf (zuletzt geprüft am: 25.06.2018)

Rensmann, L., 2004. *Demokratie und Judenbild. Antisemitismus in der politischen Kultur der Bundesrepublik Deutschland.* Wiesbaden: Verlag für Sozialwissenschaften.

Rensmann, L., 2015. *Zion als Chiffre. Modernisierter Antisemitismus in aktuellen Diskursen der deutschen politischen Öffentlichkeit.* In: Schwarz-Friesel, M. (Hrsg.), 2015. *Gebildeter Antisemitismus. Eine Herausforderung für Politik und Zivilgesellschaft.* Baden-Baden: Nomos, 93-116.

Reuters Institute. *Digital News Report 2017.* Online unter: http:// www.digitalnewsreport.org/survey/2017/overview-key-findings-2017 (zuletzt geprüft am: 25.06.2018)

Salzborn, S./Ionescu, D. (Hg.), 2014. *Antisemitismus in deutschen Parteien.* Nomos: Baden-Baden.

Schwarz-Friesel, M./Friesel, E./Reinharz, J. (Hg.), 2010. *Aktueller Antisemitismus in Deutschland. Ein Phänomen der Mitte.* Berlin, New York: de Gruyter.

Schwarz-Friesel, M./Friesel, E., 2012. „*Gestern die Juden, heute die Muslime ...*"? *Von den Gefahren falscher Analogien*. In: Botsch, G./ Glöckner, O./Kopke, C./Spieker, M. (Hg.), 2012. Islamophobie und Antisemitismus – ein umstrittener Vergleich. Berlin, Boston: de Gruyter (Europäisch-jüdische Studien. Kontroversen, Bd. 1), 29–50.

Schwarz-Friesel, M./Reinharz, J., 2013. *Die Sprache der Judenfeindschaft im 21*. Jahrhundert. Berlin, New York: de Gruyter (Europäisch-jüdische Studien – Beiträge 7).

Schwarz-Friesel, M., 2015a. *Gebildeter Antisemitismus, seine kulturelle Verankerung und historische Kontinuität: Semper idem cum mutatione*. In: Schwarz-Friesel, M. (Hg.), 2015. *Gebildeter Antisemitismus. Eine Herausforderung für Politik und Zivilgesellschaft*. Baden-Baden: Nomos, 13–34.

Schwarz-Friesel, M., 2015b. *Educated Anti-Semitism in the Middle of German Society. Empirical Findings*. In: Fireberg, H./Glöckner, O. (eds.), 2015. *Being Jewish in 21st-Century Germany*, Oldenbourg: de Gruyter, 165–187.

Schwarz-Friesel, M., 2018b. *Hass als kultureller Gefühlswert: das emotionale Fundament des aktuellen Antisemitismus*. In: Glöckner, O./Jikeli, G., (Hg.), 2018. *Das neue Unbehagen*. Hildesheim u.a.: Olms.

Schwarz-Friesel, M., 2019a. *Judenhass 2.0: Das Chamäleon Antisemitismus im digitalen Zeitalter*. In: Heilbronn et al. (Hrsg), 2019. *Neuer Antisemitismus? Fortsetzung einer globalen Debatte*. Frankfurt: Suhrkamp, 385-417.

Schwarz-Friesel, M., 2019b. *Judenhass im Internet*. Leipzig: Hentrich & Hentrich.

Schwarz-Friesel, M., 2020a. „*Wer so denkt, mordet wieder.*", Mai 2020: Gedenkrede zur Befreiung des KZ Mauthausen vor 75 Jahren. Online unter: http://www.gegendenantisemitismus. at/11052020.php.

Schwarz-Friesel, M., 2020b. *„Verbesserungsvorschläge" für Juden? – Eine gefährliche Hybris. Der Fall Mbembe aus Sicht der empirischen Antisemitismusforschung.* haGalil: https://www.hagalil.com/2020/05/mbembe-2/

Schwarz-Friesel, M. 2021. *Israelbezogener Antisemitismus und der lange Atem des Anti-Judaismus.* IDZ Jena: https://www.idz-jena.de/wsddet/wsd8-5/

Shainkman, M. (ed.) 2018. *Antisemitism Today and Tomorrow: Global Perspectives on the Many Faces of Contemporary Antisemitism.* Boston: Academic Studies Press (Antisemitism Studies).

Stopantisemitismus.de; https://www.stopantisemitismus.de/

Trachtenberg, J., 1943. *The Devil and the Jews. The Medieval Conception of the Jew and its Relation to Modern Antisemitism.* New Haven.

Weiß, M., 2021. *Zionismus als Chiffre. Der Berliner Al Quds-Marsch als Artikulationsort für Antisemitismus.* Audiatur: https://www.audiatur-online.ch/2021/04/22/zionismus-als-chiffre-der-berliner-al-quds-marsch-als-artikulationsort-fuer-antisemitismus/.

Wistrich, R., 1992. *Antisemitism: The longest hatred.* London.

Wistrich, R. S., 2010. *A Lethal Obsession: Anti-semitism from Antiquity to the Global Jihad.* New York: Random House.

Chapter Seven

Anti-Semitism: The Traps of Definitions[1]
Natan Sznaider

*Being Jewish is for me one of the undoubted facts of my
life and I have never wanted to change such facts. Such an
attitude of fundamental gratitude for what is, as it is, given
and not made, physei and not nomoi is pre-political....*

Hannah Arendt

Can, indeed may, there be a detached sociological view of anti-Semitism? Can anti-Semitism as a topic be discussed at all beyond political attributions? In the political view, the anti-Semites are always the others; the accusation of anti-Semitism often serves as a political and ideological lightning rod. Not only the reactions to the anti-Semitic attack in Halle in October 2019 have shown this clearly once again. The sociological view, however, enables us to get to the bottom of the matter. It is both further away and closer at the same time; it confronts us with the diversity of the most varied descriptions of the same reality.

Anti-Semitism, whether a feeling, a resentment, an attitude, a rumor, or even just a stereotype or prejudice about a particular social and cultural group called Jews, is part of global modernity. Anti-Semitism does not produce an incongruity of modernity that can be remedied by enlightenment. Anti-Semitism is part of the Enlightenment. And I will further discuss why this is so. And who are these Jews who are resented so

---

[1] The essay is based on a lecture given at the University of Heidelberg, July 2021. More extensively in Christian Heilbronn, Doron Rabinovici, and Natan Sznaider, Neuer Antisemitismus? Continuation of a Global Debate, Berlin: Suhrkamp, 2019.

much? So who are we talking about and theorizing about when we talk and think about these people? Are they concrete people who were born Jewish? Or are Jews and Jewesses metaphors and stand for something else?

The memory of the Holocaust had delegitimized hatred of Jews for a long time for a large part of the population. The resentment never disappeared, of course, but one had to work like the archaeologists, namely to uncover what was hidden and to make the "uncanny," the Jew, secret. So the "sinister" Jew is back, accompanied by the even more sinister Muslims. So, in the image of Europe, is the true Jew still the non-Jew, just as the true Black is the non-Black, or the true Muslim is the non-Muslim?

As historians and theorists of anti-Semitism, we are always caught in the trap of the subject matter itself. If anti-Semitism means harboring negative feelings and opinions against a collective, then analysts of anti-Semitism must address the basic collective assumptions of anti-Semitic feeling in part to decode them. It is, after all, the anti-Semites who view Jews as Jews and not as people per se. Anti-Semitism and anti-anti-Semitism always go involuntarily hand in hand in these theoretical conceptions.

As analysts of anti-Semitism, what should we do about this finding? Should we construct a theory of anti-Semitic attitudes that is completely independent of Jewish behavior or action? One speaks too readily and also too hastily about an anti-Semitism without Jews. Must Jews be seen as passive victims of resentment and hatred against them in order to arrive at a proper theory? Can such a construction work at all?

Those who talk about anti-Semitism usually find themselves caught in a fatal dichotomy between alarmists and deniers. Alarmists see the ugly face of anti-Semitism resurgent and see almost every expression of political criticism directed against Israel as a continuation of anti-Semitism by other means. Alarmists also question our everyday security and make us doubt that we live in an existentially safe world. Deniers, on the other hand, try to defend the attacks on Israel as politically justified. They deny that there is a new wave of anti-Semitism; they claim that Islamophobia is actually worse. Both sides often get lost in a debate about the legitimacy of criticizing Israel. It ends up being a discussion that reinforces the political attitudes of the speakers - one is either for or against Israel. If anything, they tend to talk about current manifestations of Islamophobia, pitting one sentiment against the other. Deniers also doubt the felt everyday experience of Jews and Jewesses. Don't exaggerate, they say, we live in the best world ever for Jews.

I would like to illustrate this with some pictures.

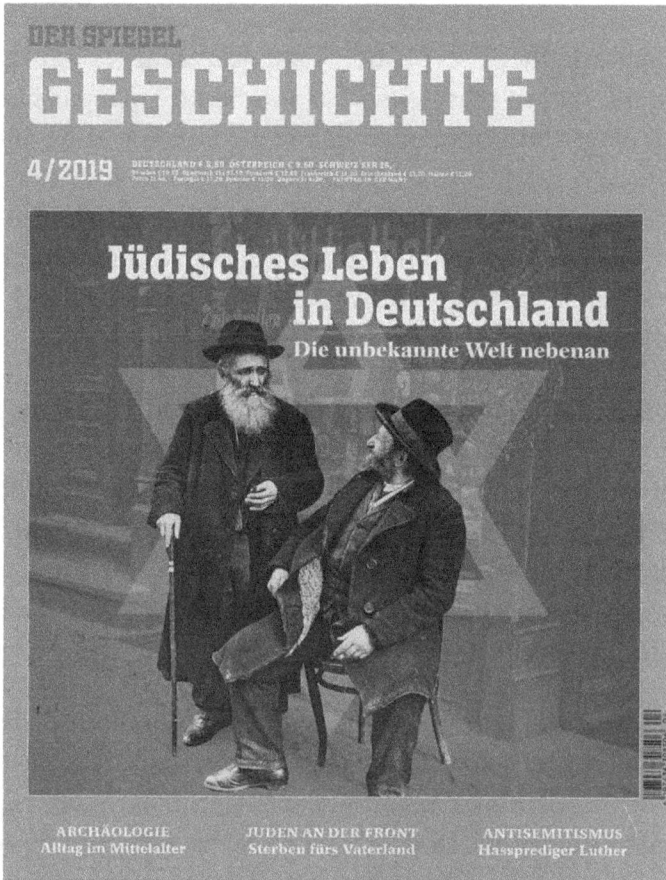

This image was a cover of a 2019 Spiegel special issue. An image from the 1920s Berlin barn district, probably immigrants from Eastern Europe. Certainly not the majority of Jews in Germany today, but they are visibly recognizable Jews. Many of the just scaffolding Jewish reactions to the photo are typical of anti-anti-Semitism.

For example, the president of the Central Council of Jews, Josef Schuster, shares,

> *"With the cover photo, Spiegel unfortunately serves up stereotypes of Jews. Especially in Germany, you hardly ever meet Jews who look like the two men in the photo."*[2]

Let's now leave aside why one hardly meets any more Jews in Germany who look like the two men in the photo. Nor is it necessary to go into the sentence "The unknown world next door", the rejection of which means at the same time that the Jewish world is supposed to be known.[3] This, of course, is also what the definition of anti-Semitism and simultaneous anti-anti-Semitism is about. Jews are supposed to look like all other people. This raises the question of why there was so much outrage from the Jewish side about this photo. Why are visibly recognizable Jews stereotyped? Does this mean that invisible Jews therefore serve the opposite of stereotype or prejudice, that is, they are true and authentic Jews? These are really not quibbles; they are key questions that go to the heart of modern societies. And this question goes to the heart of the Enlightenment and the role that Jews played in it.

---

[2] This is what Josef Schuster, chairman of the Central Council of Jews in Germany, said in Die Welt, Aug. 02, 2019

[3] The WDR started a program called "Freitagnacht Jews" in June 2021. Also the English connotation wants to transport something youthful and hip about Jews and Jewish women, to give the impression that Jews are actually like other people, just a little more.

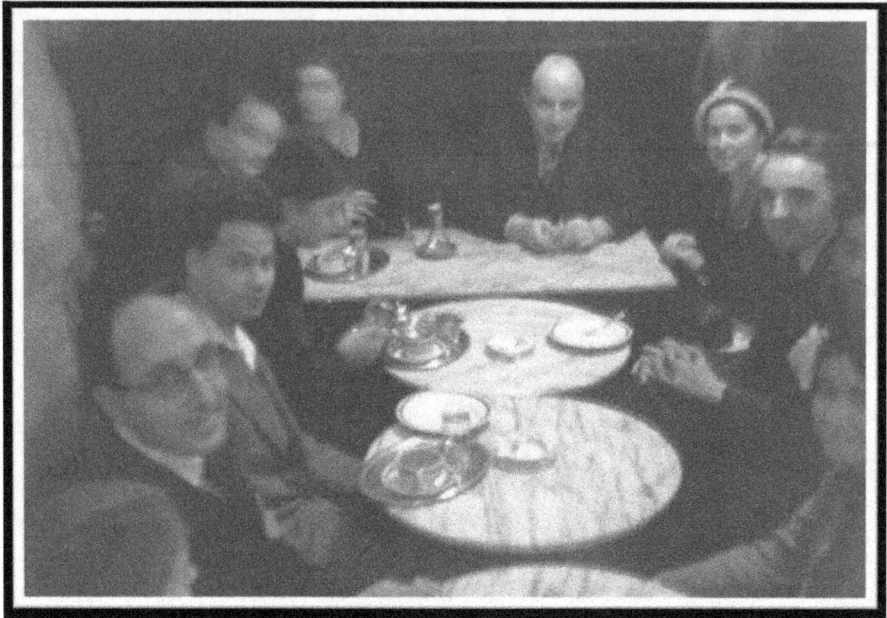

Now let's take a closer look at the next photograph. Taken in 1932 probably shortly before the election success of the NSDAP. We see the Hungarian-German-Jewish sociologist Karl Mannheim at the head of the table, around him sits his assistant Norbert Elias, Nina Rubinstein and other students. Most of them Jews and Jewish women. A pictorial document of an iconic nature. The end of an era without the participants knowing it. An eerie image indeed precisely because of the Jewish invisibility and confidence of the image. Here the Jews are invisible as such. Only the destructive anti-Semitism made them "visible" Jews. They had their experience with universalism when they began to assimilate. It was the attempt to look, to speak, to write, to be like the others, the non-Jews. In the name of a superior idea - belonging to the nation or even, in its idealistic exaltation, to the community of the enlightened. But they were not granted this affiliation; again and again they were pushed back to the particularity of their Jewishness. A year later, almost none of them were left in Germany. They had fled to France, England, Italy, the USA and Palestine.

Israel and anti-Semitism

There is also a political visibility of the Jews. The establishment of the State of Israel as an expression of Jewish political sovereignty does not make it easier for us to think about anti-Semitism. It is a global phenomenon, which of course has different connotations in Germany. Why is there so much criticism of Israel? Is the criticism justified? Is it too much criticism and the critics' motivation questionable, i.e. anti-Semitic? Does the sovereign state of Israel, with its state institutions of exercising power, play the role of the stranger in the bourgeois societies of the 19th and 20th centuries? These are, of course, questions that defy a quick answer if one does not want to fall into the shallowness of the debate over the legitimacy of criticism. After 1945, it seemed more than natural that only Zionism could reassemble what had been shattered for the Jews by the Nazis. A basic mystical event translated politically, namely to give the Jews a state. To turn a stateless people into a people with a state and a homeland, and to make Jews feel that Zionism, which was only one of the various political alternatives for Jews between the wars, turned out to be the only possible political alternative for Jews living after 1945.

The language of Israel's Declaration of Independence explains itself so clearly:

> *The catastrophe that befell the Jewish people in our time, destroying millions of Jews in Europe, irrefutably proved anew that the problem of Jewish homelessness must be solved by the restoration of the Jewish state in the Land of Israel, in a state whose gates are open to every Jew, and which secures for the Jewish people the rank of an equal nation in the family of nations.[4]*

---

[4] For the text of the Israeli Declaration of Independence, see: https://embassies. gov.il/berlin/AboutIsrael/Dokumente%20Land%20und%20Leute/Die_ Unabhaengigkeitserklaerung_des_Staates_Israel.pdf

It is a politically secular and at the same time a theologically sacred language. Immediately after the founding of the state in 1948, the chief rabbis of Israel had called a new prayer into the world: "The Prayer for the Peace of the State of Israel". It reads, "Our Heavenly Father, Rock of Israel and its Redeemer, bless the State of Israel, the beginning of the flowering of our redemption." If Israel is indeed the beginning of Jewish redemption, then criticism of Israel's political actions must at the same time be criticism of that redemption. And in addition to the theological dimension of Israel, the newly established state of Israel began with an ethnic definition of its nation and attempted, indeed had to attempt, to create a national unity out of the plurality of Jewish diaspora existence. What was heterogeneous by definition, namely Jewish diaspora existence, was now to become homogeneous. Zionism was the political answer to anti-Semitism. Therefore, the two concepts are intertwined. The concept of the sovereignty of the Israeli state clearly challenged the Jewish vision of life in the Diaspora. And this is where the critique of Israel as a European ethnonational, if not colonial, project begins. It is first and foremost a critique of the exercise of Jewish political state sovereignty. And it is a critique of the Zionists' violent seizure of land. For the idea of a state for Jews in the Middle East could only be imposed by force. The idea of a "Jewish state" - a state in which Jews and the Jewish religion have privileges from which non-Jewish citizens are often excluded - is difficult for many critics who do not want to understand Israel either theologically or historically from the Jewish situation. What seems to be the case with all, however, is that all participants in the debate employ the rhetoric of suspicion: The accusation of anti-Semitism is based on the presumption that *what is said is not what is meant*. So how to decipher when the "anti-Semite" or the "anti-Semite" claims not to be one?

The different definitions

These different sensitivities came to the fore once again in March 2021. Amid debates over the "true" nature of anti-Semitism, a group of Jewish and non-Jewish scholars issued a statement defining anti-Semitism in a way that this redefinition can be consistent with progressive politics. Since the initiative for this statement came from the Jerusalem Van Leer Institute, it was then called the *Jerusalem Declaration on Anti-Semitism.*[5] As the authors emphasize, it is written in the spirit of the Universal Declaration of Human Rights, i.e. an attempt to explain the phenomenon of anti-Semitism in general and not in particular terms. In the first article, anti-Semitism is subordinated to racism, and in a later part, a clear distinction is made between anti-Semitism and anti-Zionism, and boycotts are described as legitimate resistance that is not necessarily anti-Semitic. And literally, Article 13 states:

Therefore, comparing Israel, albeit controversially, to historical examples including settler colonialism or apartheid is not per se anti-Semitic.

In doing so, the authors submit to a particular political view of anti-Semitism, racism, and (anti)Zionism. Although the statement emphasizes that it was prepared by a large group of scholars, it is not, of course, a scientific definition of anti-Semitism.

Nor does it claim to be, but rather serves as a political rebuttal to a definition of anti-Semitism that is rejected by the authors here. This definition, the so-called IHRA (International Holocaust Remembrance Alliance, an intergovernmental body founded in 1998) definition of anti-Semitism from 2016 is the real bogeyman of the "Jerusalem Declaration."[6]

---

[5] For the German wording see: https://jerusalemdeclaration.org/wp-content/uploads/2021/03/JDA-deutsch-final.ok_.pdf

[6] For the German wording see tps://www.holocaustremembrance.com/de/node/196

This definition, too, is of course not scientific, but a political declaration, a thesis on the Jerusalem antithesis. The so-called IHRA working definition is very Israel-centric, seeing anti-Semitism and hostility to Israel as mutually constituting phenomena. Seven of its eleven examples of anti-Semitism relate directly to Israel. This working definition then becomes the basis for how many states officially define anti-Semitism. This was the case for the German government's Commissioner for Jewish Life and the Fight Against Anti-Semitism, who issued an official statement advocating that the IHRA become the basis for state action on issues of anti-Semitism.

The IHRA definition begins with the words, *"Anti-Semitism is a particular perception of Jews that may be expressed as hatred toward Jews."*

The problem with both definitions is that the object of their description remains obscure. The IHRA definition speaks of *"a particular perception of Jews"* while the Jerusalem Declaration declares right in Article 1, *"It is racist to essentialize."* Is that even true? Is it racist to essentialize? If indeed it is, then who is the Jew or Jewess that the two definitions speak of. It is the same with the IHRA. Is it indeed anti-Semitic to have a certain perception of Jews? Why should one not have certain perceptions of Jews? On July 14, 2021, the Israeli foreign minister gave a speech at the "Global Forum on Combatting Antisemitism," where he acknowledged, on the one hand, that antisemitism can go further than hatred of Jews, but at the same time committed himself to the IHRA definition. Lapid caused a great deal of turmoil in Israeli debates in July and August 2021 about how now to understand anti-Semitism. It did not add much to the understanding of even the phenomenon. What are these two definitions actually about? To equate anti-Semitism with racism has, of course, to equate the Holocaust with colonialism.

The moral narratives of the 20th century: the Holocaust and colonialism.

There are two major moral narratives of the 20th century. Israel and the Jews are in the burning mirror of both. One is the Holocaust and the historical consequence for Jews who see Israel as the guarantor of their security. Here, the establishment of the State of Israel indeed serves as redemption. But there is also another 20th century moral narrative where the Holocaust does not play a central role. Here the focus is on the atrocities of the West against the world outside the West. Not Holocaust, but colonialism and imperialism are the semantic markers in this narrative. In this narrative, Israelis are white settlers, Israel is a settler society that subjugates the indigenous population and is seen as a handout to the West. To be sure, these two moral narratives cannot be clearly separated; they are intertwined in historiography as well as in political approaches. In the Middle East conflict in particular, they are superimposed. This colonialist narrative, which was initially hardly noticed in the West, has arrived in Europe especially in recent years through immigration and global media and competes with the narrative of the Holocaust.

In the German memory space, calls for boycotts against Israel (and thus Jews) are connoted differently and thus immediately call anti-Semitism officers onto the epistemological playing field. If the knowledge frame is "colonialism," then Israelis are white settlers and the Arab population is people exploited by the colonialists, whose exploitation and exclusion is based on race. These are interest-driven political debates, not scientific ones. These arguments stem from a critical political semantics committed to emancipation and universalism, precisely the opposite knowledge structures of Zionism, which springs from the critique of emancipation and universalism. That the counter-movement is also particular is often overlooked. Rather, it is about the nexus of Enlightenment, Jews, and Israel.

Anti-Semitism and Enlightenment

Critics of Israel are very clear. Zionism and Israel deny the universalizing impulse of emancipation. Again, they are about visibility. Indeed, they do, for like postcolonialism, Zionism arose from a critique on the universal claims of enlightenment and emancipation. For Jews (and not only Jews), the motto of emancipation was: be a Jew at home and a man in the world. Emancipation demanded the public invisibility of Jews. Emancipation marked the beginning of the "invisible" Jew, who could be like all other people through the promise of citizenship. At a time when modernity also meant the transition from "community" to "society," this became an indictment of Jews. They were still a close-knit community, thus undermining the general claims of citizenship, but at the same time taking advantage of the increasing privatization and commercialization of society, this was the opinion of those who saw Jews as enemies of the nation. Jews were caught in a double bind. They were seen as too particular to be universal citizens and too universal, transcending the boundaries of citizenship, actually too cosmopolitan to be particular citizens. Thus, a few decades after the French Revolution, Karl Marx (1843) reflected in his writing "On the Jewish Question" on the political emancipation of the Jews and why it had to fail. Marx did not believe that the Jewish problem could be solved by legal means. Equal citizenship was not the problem that capitalism was. "The social emancipation of the Jew is the emancipation of society from Jewry," he wrote, and this statement became a rallying cry not only for the enemies of the Jews but also for the Jews themselves, who saw in socialism a centuries-old Jewish longing for salvation, now called "human emancipation." For in this political view, it was no longer a matter of emancipation of Jews, but of emancipation of human beings. Jews as Jews undermined this universal claim of becoming human. Particular Jews belonged to the past, had to be "improved" in order to become human beings. Thus Marx placed Jews at the center of the European drama of modernity to this day. The Jews became the symbol of all modern paradoxes. As figures of particularity, they undermined the universal aspirations of the Enlightenment. They became outsiders to the Enlightenment, still living in fantasy worlds of tight-knit communities.

Unorthodox

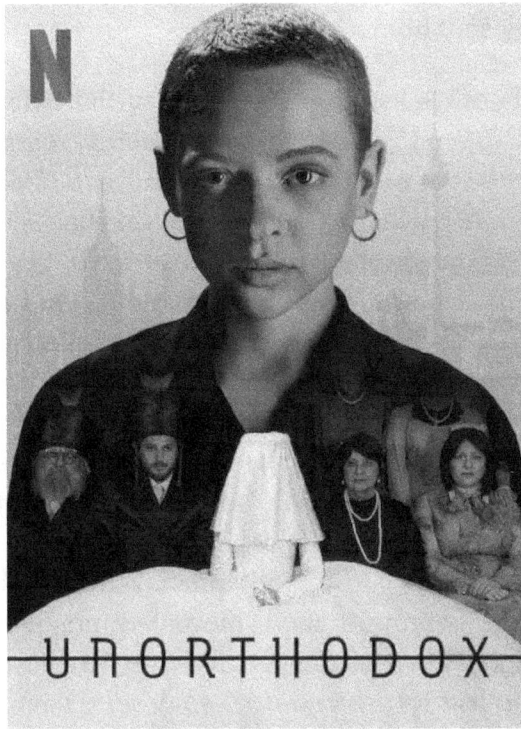

A good example of this is a German-international four-part miniseries that has been available on Netflix since March 2020. "Unorthodox" its name. Actually an emancipation story of a young woman from an ultra-Orthodox family in Brooklyn. Esty "escapes" to Berlin, where she finds a cosmopolitan group of young male and female musicians, befriends them, and ends up liberating herself both sexually and artistically. The key scene is a "rebaptism" in the Wannsee, where she throws her wig - a sign of married Jewish Orthodox women - into the water and swims in the lake with her arms crossed. After that, the path to the Berlin nightclub scene is open, plus a fulfilling sexual experience with a young Berlin musician, reconciliation with her formerly Orthodox mother who is in a couple relationship with a German woman, and insights into her self-discovery as a singer in cosmopolitan Berlin. It is this Berlin that in the end rescues the young Jewess from the particularistic clutches of the ultra-Orthodox. The Jews and Jewesses, who were wrong from the start and are portrayed as oppressors of female sexuality and free ways of life, were put in their place by the city of Berlin and its cosmopolitan citizens and in the end literally sent home.[7]

So what is it about? Is Esty representative of the state of Israel? Can it be that this dilemma of visible particularity versus "invisible" universalism, brought to life by the French Revolution, also applies to Israel today? A particularist state par excellence, a state of the Jews or even a Jewish state that defines itself beyond the post-national zeitgeist. Israel defines itself ethnically and the criteria for their citizenship as well as the criteria for their collective memory are particular, meaning that the Holocaust is commemorated as a crime against the Jewish people and not as a crime against humanity. In the series "Unorthodox," it is the pious Jews who remind Esty of the Nazi crimes. Other notions of citizenship and memory would require Israel to abandon the ethnic basis by which it defines its nationals, which is itself a historical response to anti-Semitism. When Jews were accused of being a nation within a nation, they were unable to escape this dilemma. The more Jews assimilated, the "less" they were Jews. But if one continues to feel Jewish and does so despite having assimilated, then it is a sign that one is not fully assimilated after all. And it seems that this issue also applies to Israel, which may be unable to create universal criteria of belonging. Israel defines itself as both democratic and Jewish, so its universality is inherently limited.

Anti-Semitism or not, there are clearly critics of Israel who reject the notion of a "Jewish state" (i.e., an ethnic state in which Jews enjoy privileges). These critics also attack Israel for its willingness to engage in military action and constant readiness for war. But Israel's self-image is also, of course, sovereignty, which naturally means a willingness to use force. This is also the background for Israel's insistence on its sovereignty in opposition to international legal rules and regulations. This opposition is always openly acted out when

---

[7] The Netflix series "Unorthodox" can certainly be seen as a contrast to the Israeli series "Shtissel" (also available on Netflix), which tries to follow the life of an Orthodox Jewish family in Jerusalem, without immediately pointing an enlightened finger at these Orthodox Jews.

Israel is accused of violating human rights and international law because Israel claims to insist on its sovereignty. Here, too, one should consider the historical background. In the Israeli collective memory, the failure of international law, which failed miserably for the Jews during the Holocaust and could not provide for their protection, stands out. This is one of the reasons why Israeli sovereignty is not committed to international jurisdiction. And this is where political problems that help determine political action begin.

Zionism is not the same as Judaism. In Israel, Judaism is no longer a "spaceless" religion, but a people with a land and space that must act politically. Jews in Israel have political freedom that Diaspora Jewry cannot claim for itself and therefore often relied on international protections. The establishment of the State of Israel was to fundamentally change Jewish life. Israeli Jews were to exhibit "normal" behavior. Once Jews had a home, they were to lose their foreignness and participate as political equals of world civilization. This is often not accepted. There is still an expectation that Jews should have acted more nobly than Europeans and others because of their past. There is an expectation that Israel should have avoided chauvinism and militarism, that Jews in Israel should be perfect democrats, as if state and political action were even possible that way. And this in a hostile environment that cannot and will not accept the exercise of Jewish political sovereignty. This is also the challenge to the political theory of Machiavelli, who always pointed out that the definition of "normality" in political behavior involves violence and the exercise of violence. If Jews become normal - as defined in the conventional Zionist concept of normalization - is it reasonable to expect them to form an ideal political society and act unhistorically or more morally than others? This is a dilemma that the State of Israel has not, indeed could not, solve. The realization of political normalcy and freedom by Jews, as expressed in Israel's daily behavior, is deeply offensive to many Jews and non-Jews. It is not surprising, therefore, that coverage of Israel is unbalanced. This is not necessarily anti-Semitic, but can be explained from the history of anti-Semitism. It would be surprising if this coverage were balanced. It is clear that Israel is measured and judged differently than other nation-states. Israel, in its present form, cannot expect to be treated like all other nations, since Jewish existence in and outside Israel is not comparable to the existence of other groups. This must lead to conflict. The conflict between assertions that call for a normal life for Jews and those who believe Jews should be elevated and above politics is part of this discourse. This is also what I believe is behind the BDS movement's extreme criticism of Israel. BDS stands for "Boycott, Divestment and Sanctions," a global movement that calls for cultural, academic and general boycotts against Israel. It was launched in 2005 by various Palestinian organizations. In recent years, it has become a rallying movement for the struggle against Israel. Here, once again, the previously mentioned dichotomies converge. For the friends of Israel, it is considered anti-Semitic, for the enemies of Israel rather anti-colonialist. For many, this boycott movement is an anti-Semitic phenomenon, because it is argued that BDS does not only target the state institutions of the State of Israel, does not only call for a trade ban against Israeli companies, and does not only boycott all products from Israel, but also repeatedly demands the breaking off of all contact with Israel and the Israelis. Of course, one can say that this is anti-Semitism transferred to Israel, and it may even be true, but I think one is making things too easy for oneself. There is more to it than that: on the one hand, humanitarian thought and feeling should be universal, impartial, independent, and neutral. These principles also exist in Israel, of course, but they have different connotations. Belonging to the nation-state is the normal case, and it is this normal case that, before the establishment of the State of Israel, was to make the situation for Jews who were considered not to belong in their states, and for many stateless Jews fleeing, a situation of annihilation. The human rights policy that began after World War II and specifically focused on the rights of individuals and not only on the protection of minorities is the response to the boundless failure of nation-state oriented international law, which lost its innocence, forfeited its legitimacy in the catastrophic history of the 20th century.

This is also the Jewish experience that shapes the Israeli state. Jews in particular experienced the "boundless" failure of international law during their persecution and extermination during World War II, but the consequences they drew for the Jewish state of Israel from the failure of international agreements are not aimed at delegitimizing the nation-state, but conversely at sovereignty and the military ability to defend itself. Power and the exercise of power, as well as political violence, are viewed quite positively in Israel. This complicates debates about Israel and anti-Semitism. One can, of course, continue to dream of turning swords into plowshares, just as one can dream of a world without anti-Semitism. It is a prophetic vision of world repair.

So how could there not be resentment against the Jews and their embodiment of ambivalence? Why should it be at all surprising when Jewishness, even its nation, is demonized as a symbol of Western supremacy, to be the real agent behind migration, the waves of flight, indeed the multicultural reality in the age of globalization par excellence? Why fight anti-Semitism at all, if it can be called such a widespread, global, almost common and - as Isaiah Berlin says in the sentence quoted at the beginning - necessary reaction? The answer is probably because anti-Semitism is the hatred of the universal and the particular of modern human existence. It is not just a Jewish problem, but a threat to plurality in the global age itself. The dream of perfect assimilation is an irredeemable illusion. This circumstance defines the paradoxical situation not only of Jews, but of all modern people: It is both a burden and a dignity.

Chapter Eight

Resurrection of Old Ghosts?
76 Years Later
Michael Wolffsohn

In which year are we living?
Ladies and Gentlemen
in 1348 or anno domini 2021?

Why do I ask? No, I have not mixed up the manuscript. I am not (yet) so old-fashioned that I cannot distinguish what I have experienced from what I have read. I know ("even") that we do not live in the Middle Ages today. But. Yes, but: What I, like all of you, experience, hear, see and hear, reminds me not infrequently of the Black Death, i.e. the plague pandemic, yes pandemic and not "just" epidemic, of the years 1348 to 1353. 25 million people died at that time, about a third of the world's population. And - "of course" - "the Jews were to blame". They would have poisoned the wells of good Christian people or placed poisonous mixtures elsewhere. Sounds somehow familiar and up-to-date. Doesn't it? Against, in the sense of against, thus against all facts today, again this nonsense is spread and, worse still, often believed.

In vain factual enlightenment, books, articles, lectures, seminars at universities or wherever, costly tolerance programs, weeks of brotherhood. Brotherhood? Nebbich!

In vain the fact that Jews, especially Orthodox Jews - think of Brooklyn, New York, or Mea Schearim and Bnei Brak in Israel - were coronainfied far more often than non-Jews or non-religious Jews. To all intents and purposes, therefore, "the" Jews do not qualify as a malicious viral vector against other people. At the beginning of the pandemics, Israel, measured by the number of inhabitants, climbed to the sad number 1 of the world's corona infected. No matter, "the Jews are to blame" and would be therefore to be punished. Of course, this is not the opinion of the majority, let alone all, but too many. Then Israel became vaccination world champion and number 1 in the (hopefully permanent) overcoming of the pandemic. "Clear case": "Pfizer and Moderna - firmly in Jewish hands". As ever.

How are the too-many to be re-educated? In vain, in vain, much, though not all, in vain. In vain, too, the enlightening humanity of a Lessing. In his "*Nathan,*" which premiered in 1783 and remains one of the most frequently performed plays in Germany, Lessing satirizes the anti-Judaism of the Jerusalem patriarch. To every argument exculpating "them" and the Jew, that witless Christian clergyman stereotypically retorts, "Do nothing, the Jew will be burned." T

Unbelievable, but true: Like in 1348, anti-Semitic nonsense is not only spread, but applauded. Not only by little Erna and little Moritz. On July 6, 2016, Palestinian President Mahmoud Abbas served up the age-old, medieval legend of Jewish well poisoners before the European Parliament. This time, the actors were not Jews of the Middle Ages, but contemporary Israeli rabbis. The latter, a week before his speech, had demanded that their government poison the water of Palestinians in the West Bank. At the end of Abbas' speech: standing ovation from the democratically elected European parliamentarians for that anti-Semitic filth, yes, filth. Fake News. Not "Made in America" by Donald Trump, but by the Palestine president, believed and applauded by top Europeans.

It gets even better, read: worse, actually unbelievable - but true. I am not quoting from a post of the AfD, NPD, the Reichsbürger or other alt-new-righters, I am quoting from a travel warning of the Foreign Office of the Federal Republic of Germany for the "Palestinian Territories", retrieved on October 26, 2020: "The groundwater" in the Gaza Strip "is considered polluted". A reason for the polluted groundwater is given in the introduction: "As part of the Israeli military operation "Protective Edge", heavy attacks were carried out on targets in the Gaza Strip with many deaths and injuries. This included damage to public infrastructure, such as roads, electricity, and sewage systems." The Israeli military action Protective Edge took place in the summer of 2014. in response to sustained rocket fire on Israel by Palestinian militant groups. In plain English, our State Department's verbiage says, "The Jews are to blame." Even if it were true with regard to Gaza groundwater, the German government, above all the Foreign Ministry, could have ensured that the quality of Gaza's groundwater was improved or that alternatives were provided. Moreover, it is not only since 2014 that German millions have been flowing to Hamas in the Gaza Strip. Instead of remediating the groundwater, however, Hamas preferred to produce rockets that continually rained down on Israelis.

"Protective Edge", 69 years after, July 2014.Berlin, Kurfürstendamm. Al-Kuds Day. Palestinians, fired up by mostly leftist "bio-Germans," demonstrate and chant, "Slaughter the Jews!" Or "Burn, Jew!" Or "Jew, Jew, cowardly pig ...". Or "Hamas, Hamas, Jews to the gas, Jews to the gas!" These insults of Jews, Jewish Germans, they are not incitement of the people, says the Berlin public prosecutor's office. No, not at all. May 2021: Muslims shout "Shit Jews, shit Jews!", their left-wing extremist friends look on approvingly. The alliance of Islamolinks. 1348, 2014, 2020, 2021 or not to speak of 1933. At that time "only" bio-German, today German-diverse. Result of misunderstood tolerance, which led to militancy.

Not only 76 years "after": Violence against Jews has long been part of New German everyday life. Violence in word and deed. Not only since 2020 at the Hamburg synagogue, 2019 at the Halle synagogue, the bullying in schools, on streets or in public transport, the murder of Jewish publisher Shlomo Lewin in 1980, the Munich Olympic massacre by Palestinian terrorists against Israelis in 1972, the arson attack on the Jewish old people's home in Munich as well as the murder of El Al passengers at Munich's Riem airport in 1970, or the bomb attack by left-wing terrorist Kunzelmann against The Jewish Community Center in West Berlin.

Attacks on rabbis and other people recognizable as Jews, as well as many less generally known outrages long forgotten by most, have been a scandalous routine for years, and today more than ever. The perpetrators change. 'Sometimes it is the old, resurrected right-wing ghosts, 'sometimes left-wing, 'sometimes Islamists, sometimes secular Arab terrorists. All of them alive and kicking. No way, ghosts. Monsters! Victims are and remain Jews, the perpetrators change.

On the official side, the reactions are always the same. From the Federal President to the village leader: "Not an isolated case," "Never again will we allow anti-Semitism in Germany," "More education about Nazi crimes is necessary," "Better democracy education," and so on and so forth. These proclamations and proposals make sense, but at best they are only additional measures. They do not guarantee security in the sense of physical integrity.

Lip service and appeals are no substitute for diagnosis and certainly no substitute for therapy. Those who make false findings cannot successfully heal. However, this happens all too often. The reasons for this lie deeper than the superficial empty words of those who are rightly and quite sincerely outraged might suggest. Their words are quickly blown away by the wind, and new misdeeds follow. Why? Because outrage is not enough to cure pandemics like anti-Semitism. It is considerably older than Corona 2020/21 or the Black Death of 1348. The 14th century B.C. of ancient Egypt is where the beginnings of the anti-Semitism pandemic lead. But I am not talking about antiquity or the Middle Ages, but about our present.

Liberation? Oh yes, from today's perspective. From the point of view of today's rulers and most opponents in the federal and state governments. Not all opponents, of course. Liberation was always from the point of view of Jews.

Keyword "language". School wisdom says that the prerequisite and decisive instrument for successful integration is mastery of the national language. In our case, that means German. Let's look back: Did Heinrich Heine not know German? Or Kurt Tucholsky etc. etc.?

Were they successfully integrated?

Like almost all Jews living in Germany, the President of the Central Council, Dr. Josef Schuster, even I, as a German professor, have a command of the German language, both written and spoken. If the aforementioned school wisdom were true, we would not have to talk about anti-Semitism here and now. What do we learn from it? That some of the basic assumptions about integration in general and anti-Semitism in particular are unfortunately wrong.

Equally wrong is the school wisdom that anyone who can speak German and is not a burden on the German social security system will be easily integrated. Hardly any Jew was or is a burden to German social security funds. But we still have to fight the anti-Semitism virus.

Equally wrong is this school wisdom: minorities who do not drop bombs on the majority society are integrated effortlessly. Have you heard anywhere that Jews in Germany throw bombs at anyone or would be a security risk?

Conversely, however, Jews live insecurely. Still or already again in Germany. Not only in Germany, but in Europe in general, especially in the supposedly so enlightened, liberal and exemplary humane, cosmopolitan West of Europe. Security personnel - everywhere in front of and in Jewish institutions of Western Europe and Germany. Few like to hear it, but it is true: In Victor Orban's supposedly arch-reactionary and anti-Semitic Hungary, there are no security personnel in front of Jewish institutions. It is not needed. Not even in front of Budapest's main synagogue.

France has seen some 100,000 Jews leave in the last twenty years. Most of them went to Israel. In France they are free, but no longer safe. In Israel they are free and safe. Are we Jews safe in Germany? In France, Denmark, Sweden or even Great Britain, where Jews were threatened until recently by the left-wing anti-Semite Jeremy Corbyn?

Unlike 1945/1948 - Israel today is an attractive country in which to live well. Israel today offers Jews not only security of life, it also offers high quality of life. The sun shines, the summer is safe, the education system is performance-oriented, the infrastructure is excellent, Islamic and Islamist terror is now more in control than in Europe, anti-Semitism is an internal Jewish problem, and even gourmets get their money's worth. I exaggerate on purpose: For decades, Israeli restaurants offered mainly chicken, chicken, chicken and more chicken, so that in the end the guests cackled. Tempi passati. Not only does one eat well in Israel, one is safe there as a Jew. Unlike in 1933, we Jews today have a life insurance called Israel. We Jews today have an alternative, precisely this. Germany's non-Jewish majority also has an alternative: protect or lose loyal, peaceful, fluent German-speaking, well-educated, gainfully employed, tax-paying Jewish citizens who enrich the German economy and culture. We Jews have not been at the mercy of non-Jews in Germany and worldwide since 1948, since Israel has existed. We live gladly and despite known deficits well in Federal Germany, but we do not beg to be allowed to live here or even just to survive.

Back to the keyword "liberation". The Germans were liberated in 1945. They did not liberate themselves from their own criminals. My German Jewish parents and grandparents, who fled Hitler's Germany in 1939 to Palestine, felt liberated in 1945, as did all Jews. But most Germans may not have felt liberated in 1945. Today it is different. Thanks to the Federal German democracy. Today, most Germans evaluate and refer to the defeat of Hitler's Germany as liberation.

The Germans, yes, "the" Germans first and foremost owe their liberation as well as the fruits of freedom to "the" Americans. I cannot help feeling that many (too many for me) Germans resent and forget "the" Americans for their liberation to this day. Trump is just an excuse. Looked at closely, "the" Germans were liberated twice by "the" Americans in the 20th century. From the reactionary Kaiser in 1918 and from the criminal Hitler in 1945. Without America, no German democracy. Neither from 1919 to 1930/33 nor since 1949 Alt-BRD and since 1990 Neu-BRD. Today, and not only since Trump, it is part of Germany's political fashion to rail against America, to give the U.S. democracy tutoring and to act downright chutzpedick as a moral world power. More German gratitude, above all modesty, and much less anti-Americanism would be appropriate.

New German anti-Americanism and New German anti-Semitism plus anti-Israelism are closely intertwined. Long before Trump, and even under the highly sympathetic but unfortunately hapless Obama, too many Germans consider America "monster" number one and Israel "monster" number two. Israel, which a clueless former German foreign minister, following and running with the German zeitgeist, denigrated as an "apartheid state." This apartheid nonsense is often followed by the Nazi-Israel comparison. So far, this has mostly (though not always) remained outside the executive, legislative and judicial branches of government.

Let me state further facts 76 years "after".

Fact 1: Some cite neo-Nazis and other **right-wing extremists** as the main danger to Jews. On the part of the authorities, apparently irrefutable figures are presented for this. It is the numbers that are disputed, not this danger. It is undeniable. Instead of arguing about it with "the" state, one should not overlook the all but non-violent hostility towards Jews of the **left-wing extremists**. Not to mention the anti-Jewish terror of **militant Muslims**. Ghosts? All of them alive and kicking. That left-wing extremist anti-Semitism is not old but new is a legend, and legends are not facts. Islamic anti-Semitism, and not only Islamist anti-Semitism, is anything but new. It is not even new in or from Germany. From 1939 to 1945 at the latest, Hitler's Germany, the Grand Mufti of Jerusalem Hadj Amin el-Husseini and the Iraqi nationalist Gailani, as well as Muslims from the Caucasus, worked together. They were united in word and deed against "the" Jews and, Husseini, even more so against the Zionists. Against the majority truly non-Zionist Jews of Serbia, Husseini mobilized Muslims in Bosnia-Herzegovina in the Holocaust. After 1945, Old Nazi fighters found benevolent reception especially in Egypt and Syria. There they helped not least the military in the fight against the Jewish State.

Fact 2: In the fight against the national German epidemic of right-wing anti-Semitism, some resort to devious medicine. For example, they want to ban the black-white-red flag of the German Empire. In doing so, they unspokenly imply that that Hohenzollern monarchy could be equated with the criminal state of the Nazis. Hohenzollern demonology is currently fashionable ideology. In the association of the German historians and (naturally) historians also its top is not immune against it. Absurd. Today's right-wing extremists are similarly absurd, i.e. clueless, albeit under different political auspices, when they wave this flag wherever. The Nazis reintroduced the imperial black-white-red in 1933 and replaced it completely from 1935 on, because "Führer" and swastika were supposed to outshine everyone and everything. The same applies to the Reich war flag, which right-wing extremists today carry like a with and in front of them. It was the war flag of the black-white-red empire. The Reich war flag of the Nazis looked different. With swastika of course. If you want to ban black-white-red, you would have to ban the Bundestag from the Reichstag. This was built from 1884 to 1894 during the black-white-red empire. One would then also have to ban the black and white jersey of the German national soccer team. Since their first international match in 1908, the German kickers have worn black and white. Black and white were the colors of Prussia. Prussia's king was German Emperor, and Prussia today is even more sinister and repulsive to many than the Empire. So, abolish it? Absurd, but with such absurdities some try to fight anti-Semitism and right-wing extremism. Nothing is gained for the safety of Jews, and the necessary fight against right-wing extremists degenerates into a farce. The crowning ridiculousness would be the desire to abolish the German language. Even for this there would be an apparent rationale: Hitler and his fellow murderers spoke German.

Fact 3: From all **three extremist groups** - right-wing, left-wing, Islamic fanatics - Jews are threatened with danger to life and limb. I repeat on purpose: The perpetrators change, not the victims.

Fact 4: Jewish victims do not care whether the violence is threatened by right-wingers, left-wingers or Islamists from within the country or abroad. **Violence is violence**, is crime, and must be punished as a crime. If the perpetrator or perpetrators are of foreign origin or belong to a non-Christian religion, the act belongs to be punished as a crime.

Fact 5: Among the standard responses is this sentence: "Hostility toward Jews goes, not only in Germany, far into the middle of society." That's right. What is meant by this in the public discussion is primarily the bourgeois-conservative, *right-wing* liberal, generally right-wing (not right-wing extremist) **part of society**. It remains to be said, however, that bourgeois, in the sense of bourgeois and citoyen, rarely, if ever, throw bombs. This applies to right-wing liberal-conservative as well as left-wing liberal bourgeois. Neither right-liberal nor left-liberal bourgeois resort to violence themselves. They do, however, justify their smarts in an unspoken way.

Fact 6: What some people often like to keep quiet about: **Hostility towards Jews goes nationally and internationally also far into the left-liberal parts of society**. One proof of many are the disputes about the activities of the apparently "only" against Israel, but in fact, as confirmed by the Bundestag 2019, directed against "the" Jews and especially successful at German and other universities **BDS campaign**. This demands a boycott of, disinvestment (end and reduction of investments) in, and sanctions (punitive measures) against Israel. "The" Jews are thereby portrayed as Israel's extended arm. Among the defenders of these derailments are mostly so-called intellectuals of left-liberal color. They themselves are not anti-Semites, but their useful idiots. Especially when they attack Felix Klein, the Federal Commissioner against Anti-Semitism, as has happened several times. In contrast to the preachers on duty, he follows up his words with deeds. His critics apparently only want inconsequential outrage as symbolic politics. That's what the city-state of Hamburg seemed to be aiming for in the fall of 2020. Instead of paid expertise in the fight against anti-Semitism, proposed by the Jewish communities, they are looking for a volunteer. With all due honor, volunteers cannot really replace full-time workers.

Symbol or paper politics also in the Bundestag. The passed with the votes from the coalition and opposition (against minorities on both sides) on May 17, 2019, a resolution that called BDS "anti-Semitic." BDS and partners should henceforth no longer receive German funds. Powerful words. They were immediately invalidated by dissenters. Norbert Röttgen (CDU) was the director. He and his colleagues succeeded in tearing down the anti-BDS wall. German money continues to flow towards BDS. Love greetings from Berlin.

In the fight against the right, one sometimes encounters a tantalizing double standard, even among left-wing liberals. Let's call it hypocrisy. I'll get specific and look at the current double standard of the S. Fischer publishing house towards the writer Monika Maron. It belongs to the Georg von Holtzbrinck publishing group. The chairman of its management board is Stefan von Holtzbrinck, the younger son of the company's founder. Dieter von Holtzbrinck is the elder son. Both branches jointly award the Georg von Holtzbrinck Prize. One is for science journalism, the other for business journalism. Both Holtzbrinck companies are based in the beautiful city of Stuttgart.

Monika Maron received the German National Prize in 2009, along with numerous other prestigious awards. Now she has been given the boot by S. Fischer Verlag. In a circular letter to the authors, the publishing management explains: S. Fischer Verlag does not want to "indirectly support a publishing context that contradicts the tradition, history and values of the publishing house." Maron is thereby expressly accused of closeness to the AfD, even to its "wing." If this were true, I, as a German-Jewish historian, son and grandson of Holocaust survivors, would never, ever defend Monika Maron. I defend her, however, because I have known and appreciated her family history "Pawels Briefe" (published by S. Fischer) since 1999, and she herself for twenty years. In "Pawels Briefe" she set a literary monument to her Jewish grandfather. A moving read, full of empathy for this Jew and "the" Jews par excellence. In the public debate about her rude expulsion, she could have effortlessly used your "Jewish Shield". She would have been immediately out of the "line of fire. She showed nobility and did not. Precisely for this reason, it is worth taking a brief look at the history of S. Fischer Verlag and, above all, at the values and tradition mentioned (but not specified) by the current management of the publishing house. The website of the GvH Group also refers to these values.

It was founded in 1886 by Samuel Fischer. Today, it is still one of the giants of German literary history. The "Jewish publishing house" was "Aryanized" from 1936, and after 1945 it was returned to Fischer's daughter and son-in-law. Both withdrew from 1963. The Georg von Holtzbrinck publishing group gradually took over the company.

Who was Georg von Holtzbrinck, whose name the publishing group still bears today and which, together with Dieter-von-Holtzbrinck-Medien (DvH), awards the prestigious Georg von Holtzbrinck Prize? On the GvH Group's website, we read: "The company's founder Georg von Holtzbrinck (*1909 - †1983) had begun with the subscription distribution of books and magazines in the 1930s". As late as the beginning of 2020, this could also be read: "We preserve and at the same time develop the great heritage of our traditional houses... We feel deeply committed to our origins and our traditional values..." Let the few, brittle facts be added:

Georg von Holtzbrinck began his entrepreneurial career in 1931, the same year he joined the Nazi Students' Association, although it was still banned at the time. At his Cologne university, that Nazi organization was "underrepresented" in 1931, writes his biographer, Thomas Garke-Rothbart ("vital for our business..." Georg von Holtzbrinck as a Publishing Entrepreneur in the Third Reich, Munich 2008). Career pressure therefore did not (yet) play a role there. It follows from this: Publisher Georg von Holtzbrinck was thus more of a Nazi precursor than a Nazi fellow traveler. He became a full member of the NSDAP on May 1, 1933, and remained so until 1945. For Georg von Holtzbrinck, the end of the Nazi dictatorship was rather bitter in business terms, because he had profited enormously from the Nazi regime. The German Labor Front and the Wehrmacht were major customers for his print products. The Nazi values were therefore economically valuable for Georg von Holtzbrinck. They laid the foundation for the company's rapid rise in publishing quality and quantity.

Georg von Holtzbrinck's biography is divided into two parts. Until 1945, he was a Nazi profiteer throughout. After 1945, his and his companies' services to West German democracy are indisputable. Does his second biography outshine the first to such an extent that Georg von Holtzbrinck is considered a role model for West Germany? Can, should, may such a personality be the namesake of prestigious prizes, even of liberal media houses? Is this the tradition, are these the values to which S. Fischer Verlag refers to Monika Maron, the granddaughter of Pawel Iglarz, who was probably murdered in the Kulmhof extermination camp in August 1942?

In the left-liberal context, I should also mention the Henry Nannen Prize for Journalists. It is named after the longtime head of "Stern" magazine. Before these long Federal German years, he served willingly and diligently as a propagandist during the planned thousand Nazi years, during the World War even in an SS propaganda company. Until 1979, he had covered that up. Neither left nor liberal. Shall I remind you of other moral icons of our New German Republic? Günter Grass, who most recently openly and vehemently attacked the Jewish state shamelessly and counterfactually? Or should I....? No, enough, you get my point.

Fact 7: Our officials in state, justice and society really want to protect the Jews. Or is this only hypocritically proclaimed to the outside world? The Minister of the Interior of Saxony-Anhalt was quoted these days from an internal meeting as saying that the Jews would be to blame if the police could no longer adequately take care of the concerns of the rest of the population because of the tightened protective measures for them. He quickly corrected this either sincere or misquoted statement. But even sincere willingness does not mean ability. The lack of ability in Germany has deep-seated causes.

One of them is explained by fact 8, which at the same time describes the deeply human and sympathetic, even lovable, nature of the

Federal Republic of Germany. Earlier German states were power-obsessed, Federal Germany is power-forgetful. Even democratically instituted and controlled violence, both internally (police) and externally (military), is actually taboo in our country. This is highly sympathetic, but unfortunately unrealistic. In our so sympathetically anti-heroic society, it has led - in addition to the neglect of the Bundeswehr - to the neglect and sometimes even the disparagement of the police. Not only by those who denigrate police officers as "pigs" or "cops," but also by some (politicians) who are protected by these same police every day from extremists of every ideology.

Fact 9: Out of an inherently sympathetic sense of freedom, our judiciary refrains from the required application of the laws that do exist for the containment of violence. In this way, the judiciary gives extremists in general (and not only in relation to Jews) the freedom to use violence.

Fact 10: As few as there are "the" Germans, there are no "the" police. Their personnel, as in any large organization, is multi-faceted. Certainly, most of them are decent citizens "like you and me" who want to safeguard the law and order of the German democracy. In addition, as we know, there are also right-wing extremists in the police. **In the police does not mean "the" police.**

Fact 11: Without snooping for opinions, the police must, indeed must, develop methods that, on the one hand, do not let extremists of any color 'in' and, on the other hand, 'kick them out'. Respect, appreciation and gratitude for the police are indispensable. The less appreciation and the more hackles the police receive, the fewer citizens "like you and me" will become police officers. Without motivation, no one can work well. Especially in Bavaria, the police get this motivation. This is one of the reasons why Munich is one of the safest cities in the world.

Anyone who, like the German organs of internal and external security, receives so little ideal and material appreciation cannot work well. The deficits of the non-anti-Semites also condition the glaring operational deficits in the fight against enemies of the Jews. Yes, they encourage the Jew-haters. In the face of rising anti-Semitism, outrage and education are good, right and important. They are not enough for security.

The old, right-wing, left-wing and Islamist ghosts are not zombies, for they are anything but will-less or bereft of their old souls. They are thoroughly resurrected. 76 years "after" they are for us Jews the three main perpetrators and also -offenders. Like most perpetrators, they have fences and useful idiots to help them. 76 years "after" most Germans have internalized the values of the Open Society. Not only we Jews, the Open Society is surrounded by three main enemies: Rightists, Leftists, Islamists. All three dispose of partly voluntarily, partly involuntarily useful idiots. The values of the Open Society are often on the defensive. So it is now. Those who want the Open Society must protect it offensively. This is 76 years "after" our common task, the task of Jews and non-Jews. Long live the Open Society of the Federal Republic of Germany.